ACCIDENTAL INTOLERANCE

ACCIDENTAL INTOLERANCE

How We Stigmatize ADHD and How We Can Stop

Susan C. C. Hawthorne

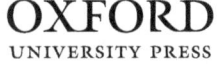
UNIVERSITY PRESS

OXFORD
UNIVERSITY PRESS

Oxford University Press is a department of the University of Oxford.
It furthers the University's objective of excellence in research, scholarship,
and education by publishing worldwide.

Oxford   New York
Auckland   Cape Town   Dar es Salaam   Hong Kong   Karachi
Kuala Lumpur   Madrid   Melbourne   Mexico City   Nairobi
New Delhi   Shanghai   Taipei   Toronto

With offices in
Argentina   Austria   Brazil   Chile   Czech Republic   France   Greece
Guatemala   Hungary   Italy   Japan   Poland   Portugal   Singapore
South Korea   Switzerland   Thailand   Turkey   Ukraine   Vietnam

Oxford is a registered trademark of Oxford University Press in the UK
and certain other countries.

Published in the United States of America by
Oxford University Press
198 Madison Avenue, New York, NY 10016

© Oxford University Press 2014

All rights reserved. No part of this publication may be reproduced, stored in a
retrieval system, or transmitted, in any form or by any means, without the prior
permission in writing of Oxford University Press, or as expressly permitted by law,
by license, or under terms agreed with the appropriate reproduction rights organization.
Inquiries concerning reproduction outside the scope of the above should be sent to the
Rights Department, Oxford University Press, at the address above.

You must not circulate this work in any other form
and you must impose this same condition on any acquirer.

Library of Congress Cataloging-in-Publication Data
Hawthorne, Susan, 1956–
Accidental intolerance : how we stigmatize ADHD and how we can stop / Susan Hawthorne.
   p. ; cm.
Includes bibliographical references.
ISBN 978–0–19–997738–3 (hardcover : alk. paper)
I. Title.
[DNLM: 1. Attention Deficit Disorder with Hyperactivity.   2. Social Stigma.
3. Social Values.   4. Biomedical Research—ethics. WS 350.8.A8]
RJ506.H9
362.19685'89—dc23
2013005494

9 8 7 6 5 4 3 2 1
Printed in the United States of America
on acid-free paper

To Grant, who has been patient.

CONTENTS

Introduction — 1
1. ADHD in Medicine — 13
2. How Science Shapes ADHD — 46
3. Social Allies and Adversaries — 79
4. Feedback: Values in ADHD Science — 115
5. Accidental Intolerance — 142
6. New Directions — 175

Index — 199

INTRODUCTION

Attention-deficit hyperactivity disorder (ADHD) is part of our cultural landscape. It's also in our genes, our neurotransmitters, and our scientific, medical, and educational institutions. It's part of the economy—said to drag it down, sapping productivity and increasing healthcare costs—but it provides enormous profits for the pharmaceutical industry. It comes as a great relief to many struggling parents and teachers, and to many adults who are diagnosed, yet strikes others as "medicalization of underperformance" (Conrad & Potter, 2000, 573) or intolerance of human variation. Most people interested in ADHD—diagnosable individuals, parents, teachers, doctors, psychologists, scientists—are concerned to ease the difficulties faced by ADHD-diagnosable people, offering support in various ways. Most wish to decrease stigmatization and to remove the moralizing tendency from our judgments of ADHD. Yet many professionals describe ADHD-associated behaviors in terms like thoughtless, ill considered, random, impulsive, and delayed in moral regulation (Barkley, 1997, 248) or emphasize morally tinged associations with the diagnosis, such as low work or academic achievement, substance abuse, or sexual acting out (Clarke, Barry, McCarthy, Selikowitz, & Johnstone, 2007; Faraone & Wilens, 2003; Hechtman et al., 2004).

Sharp differences in perspective have continued for decades. But shouldn't the "ADHD wars" be over by now, controversies put to rest, the diagnosis accepted "on a par with diabetes," as the American Psychiatric Association puts it (Anonymous, 2007)? In some ways, they *are* over. Despite long-standing arguments that ADHD is overdiagnosed, overtreated, ill-defined, driven by pharmaceutical companies, poorly understood, moralistic, pejorative, medicalizing, and so forth—despite all this, rates of diagnosis had reached approximately 9.5% among children and adolescents by 2010 (Zoler, 2010); 11% by 2012 (Centers for Disease Control and Prevention, 2012); and 4.4% among adults (Kessler et al.,

2006). Social, medical, and scientific institutions and individual lives are structured according to the diagnosis; millions of people are grateful for it, and—at least in some circles—stigma has decreased enough that diagnosed individuals make no effort to hide their ADHD status.

But widespread acceptance and the veneer of stabilized science, medicine, and social acceptance belie still-controversial data, attitudes, assumptions, and practices embedded in today's understanding of ADHD. Alongside widely accepted scientific findings remain significant knowledge gaps and open questions. Medical compassion might be widely accepted, but the economic constraints on clinical practice are less so. Some individual and social needs, interests, and attitudes are widely shared; others are contested. Such debates, gaps, and constraints present the puzzle with which I began research on the scientific, medical, and philosophical grounding of ADHD: What exactly, I wondered, keeps these controversies going? Does one side have the facts, while another obtusely denies them? Does someone have claim to an ethical high ground, while others are exploitive? I have found that there are no straightforward answers to such questions. Instead, multiple groups have contributed to today's understanding of ADHD, in all its complexity, with all its benefits and drawbacks.

The first three chapters argue that when it comes to ADHD, no one has a claim to undisputed truth or right. Medical thought and practice decides what constitutes disease; but these decisions overlook some options. Scientific practice carves out phenomena to study, choosing—from among various possibilities—what phenomena are worthy of study and how to define them. Educators and parents, alongside diagnosable adults and teens and the wider society, choose which traits and behaviors are desirable, and which are not—again, the element of choice is important. In each of these venues, participants rely both on facts as currently understood, and on institutional and personal values to make their choices. In complex ways, the choices blend a rich spectrum of facts, values, and interests to form today's understanding of ADHD and the practices surrounding it.

Recognizing the existence of options, and the blended role of fact and value, leaves us free to consider the extent to which we should endorse the facts and values associated with today's understanding of ADHD. I argue that there is an important reason we should not: In a nutshell, the combined choices have—accidentally—reinforced intolerance of ADHD-diagnosable individuals. Grouping certain human propensities into the class "ADHD" has largely been by choice, rather than a necessity. But the choices made, and the associated practices, have established a view in which ADHD is a focus of intolerance: Those who are diagnosable are marked as different—and as undesirable.

The central insight that led to this conclusion came from thinkers in philosophy of science and science studies who emphasize the inseparability of science and society. The sciences (including clinical science) and society (including clinical medicine) change in response to each other. For example, the mutual influences affect what scientists study—what facts are produced— and, in turn, the facts produced affect social interests. Taking this perspective, an aspect of the present understanding of ADHD becomes clear: It is a hybrid concept, encompassing multiple viewpoints. It is medical, focused on impairments in individuals, diagnostic criteria, and treatment possibilities. It is scientific, focused primarily on individual biology. It is social, addressing needs of schools, parents, the workplace, and affected individuals.

Thinking in these terms sets an agenda. To see the mutual influences, we need to consider and assess current views and conflicts, but we also need to see where those views came from. And we need to look not just at science, medicine, society, or diagnosable individuals but at *all* of these, considering the varying needs, interests, and forms of acceptable knowledge in each venue. Finally, we need to consider the interactions among the various venues: What does each contribute, or make problematic, in today's views of ADHD? How has the current view of ADHD come to be stabilized, in concept and practice, and what drives the continuing controversy?

First, despite its being complex and contentious, there *is* a relatively stabilized ADHD concept with which we work. Thousands of scientific, medical, education, and mass media articles are published using the concept; treatment standards exist; and conversational and attitudinal norms, although not as clear-cut as scientific/medical definitions, inform our joint discussions. Very briefly, the concept is that certain clinically identifiable patterns of behavior indicate underlying biological dysfunctions that impair affected individuals in certain situations. The behavior patterns are variable but are consistent with the lists codified by the American Psychiatric Association's *Diagnostic and Statistical Manual of Mental Disorders* (DSM; see Table I.1). The revised manual, DSM-5, like its immediate predecessors DSM-IV and DSM-IV-TR, divides ADHD into three subtypes: hyperactive-impulsive, inattentive, and combined (American Psychiatric Association, 1994; American Psychiatric Association, 2000; American Psychiatric Association, 2013).[1] The biological aspect of ADHD is not stipulated by the DSM, but, as argued in Chapters 1 and 2, is nevertheless part of the standard view. Impairments include difficulties with school work and with boring or confining adult work, difficulties with attention or

Table I.1. DSM-IV-TR Diagnostic Criteria for Attention-Deficit Hyperactivity Disorder[2]

A. Either (1) or (2):
   (1) six (or more) or the following symptoms of **inattention** have persisted for at least 6 months to a degree that is maladaptive and inconsistent with developmental level:
   Inattention
   (a) often fails to give close attention to details or makes careless mistakes in schoolwork, work, or other activities
   (b) often has difficulty sustaining attention in tasks or play activities
   (c) often does not seem to listen when spoken to directly
   (d) often does not follow through on instructions and fails to finish schoolwork, chores, or duties in the workplace (not due to oppositional behavior or failure to understand instructions)
   (e) often has difficulty organizing tasks and activities
   (f) often avoids, dislikes, or is reluctant to engage in tasks that require sustained mental effort (such as schoolwork or homework)
   (g) often loses things necessary for tasks or activities (e.g., toys, school assignments, pencils, books, or tools)
   (h) is often easily distracted by extraneous stimuli
   (i) is often forgetful in daily activities

   (2) six (or more of the following symptoms of **hyperactivity-impulsivity** have persisted for at least 6 months to a degree that is maladaptive and inconsistent with developmental level:
   Hyperactivity
   (a) often fidgets with hands or feet or squirms in seat
   (b) often leaves seat in classroom or in other situations in which remaining seated is expected
   (c) often runs about or climbs excessively in situations in which it is inappropriate (in adolescents or adults, may be limited to subjective feelings of restlessness)
   (d) often has difficulty playing or engaging in leisure activities quietly
   (e) is often "on the go" or often acts as if "driven by a motor"
   (f) often talks excessively
   Impulsivity
   (g) often blurts out answers before questions have been completed
   (h) often has difficulty awaiting turn
   (i) often interrupts or intrudes on others (e.g., butts into conversations or games)

(continued)

Table I.1. (Continued)

B. Some hyperactive-impulsive or inattentive symptoms that caused impairment were present before age 7 years.
C. Some impairment from the symptoms is present in two or more settings (e.g., at school [or work] and at home).
D. There must be clear evidence of clinically significant impairment in social, academic, or occupational functioning.
E. The symptoms do not occur exclusively during the course of a Pervasive Developmental Disorder, Schizophrenia, or other Psychotic Disorder and are not better accounted for by another mental disorder (e.g., Mood Disorder, Anxiety Disorder, Dissociative Disorder, or a Personality Disorder).

(American Psychiatric Association, 2000, 92–93).

concentration more generally, trouble in social relationships, and increased risk of additional behaviors considered problematic, such as smoking and substance abuse, and increased risk of additional mental disorders, including learning disorders, conduct disorders, and depression.

Tracing the source of today's standard views and today's objections leads back several decades. In the 1970s, before ADHD was so called, clinicians instead adopted a similar category termed "hyperkinesis." Already, critics voiced objections that drug companies were unethically promoting the diagnosis—a common concern today. People already raised worries about "labeling" or stigmatizing, and they observed the values and judgments in the DSM symptom lists. Clearly, differences in values drive such debates, but so does lack of scientific closure. Conflicting views stated in the 1970s and 1980s have continued into the present. Continued issues include lack of consensus on ADHD's causes, and disagreements over diagnostic criteria, their application, and ADHD prevalence.

Considering the sources of the predominant view, the ongoing controversies, and their consequences from a broadly philosophical viewpoint, rather than from a purely empirical, practical, or ethical perspective, reveals connections among specifics that are hard to see when one's focus is on the detail. To that end, the chapters draw on a wide range of texts, theories, and analytic methods. Sources include current views of ADHD in medicine, science, and education. In some cases, I interpret the scope of the content empirically—for example, determining the percentage of science publications that take a particular perspective toward ADHD. But much of the analysis is more theoretical, synthesizing arguments over principle, reports of attitudes and interests, and expressed views regarding goals of medicine, science, education, or parents.

Each chapter draws on standard literatures, then moves to philosophical analysis. With this strategy, readers can consider the options available in their own institutions or families, as well as those available elsewhere. So, Chapter 1, which interprets ADHD concepts and practices in medical fields, discusses current medical literature in the light of philosophical issues about disease definitions, medicalization, and dimensional versus categorical categorization. Chapter 2, on the sciences of ADHD, briefly reviews current scientific understanding of ADHD, but turns to philosophy of science to interpret scientific methodology and goals. For the discussion of interactions among medicine, science, and broader society in Chapter 3, Bruno Latour's actor-network theory provides an apt metaphor. The literatures of medical ethics and feminist philosophy of science inform Chapters 4 and 5, which demonstrate the values embedded in science and their consequences. Chapter 6 turns to American Pragmatism, updated with feminist philosophy of science, to propose new practices in science, medicine, education, and wider society to alleviate the problem of accidental intolerance.

Many readers may already be resisting the direction the analysis is heading, thinking that ADHD is a clinical necessity. After all, it has been a standardized cornerstone of treatment for decades now. Yet Chapter 1 will show that relevant controversies persist in medicine. Rather than being a simple checklist, or list of signs and symptoms, the understanding of ADHD has several layers, each of which contains contested elements. One layer is the consideration of what constitutes disease or disorder generally; another is the definition of mental (as opposed to physical) disorder generally; and a third is the DSM's definition of mental disorder. Medical models of these articulate a view in which mental disorders are biological dysfunctions in individuals, with the particular clinical criteria that they are identifiable, causally explicable, and amenable to medical treatment. As already mentioned, not all these elements are required by the DSM. This disalignment gives rise to some controversies, as does the DSM's additional criterion that mental disorders are categorical (black and white, you-have-it-or-you-don't) diagnoses—a criterion not required by a medical model. The biological and categorical features, however, address clinical needs, both in keeping focus on individuals—a physician's area of expertise and control—and in simplifying and standardizing, as much as possible at present, a complex diagnosis. In addition to these intramural debates among competing medical views, outsiders contest the categories more broadly. Medicalization of behavior, reduction of individual variation to types, the emphasis on pharmacological treatment rather than social change—these and other alternative viewpoints continue to exist despite the widespread uptake of the relatively standardized medical model of ADHD.

Other readers might resist the analysis on the grounds that the science of ADHD is the ultimate arbiter and that the sciences are clearly on the right track if not yet completely definitive. Chapter 2 explains remaining controversies among scientific experts. These, in principle, are ultimately resolvable. But the chapter also explains how current scientific methodology shapes understanding of ADHD—in choices made apart from data. Human behavior, traits, and capacities are complex, and they can be described and examined in multiple ways. The choice to study the particular complex that constitutes ADHD is guided by multiple factors in addition to findings that reinforce the existence of the phenomenon itself. Some of these factors, like the availability of funding, are sociological; these are not the subject of Chapter 2. Instead, the focus is on how the assumptions, needs, and methodologies of science reinforce a particular view of ADHD. One very basic assumption in the science is that explanations will refer only to physical (material) entities and processes involving them. Although not all research is expressly biological, this assumption aligns with aspects of the medical view of mental disorders, placing the emphasis in biology, just as is the case in medicine. In another example, today's sciences need cross-disciplinary data convergence. To achieve this, scientists in diverse fields must employ similar definitions or operationalizations for phenomena of interest. Models of ADHD must then be consonant with other areas of science, limiting the range of acceptable hypotheses. Similarly, methodological concerns require consistency in data comparisons among studies of ADHD, tending to reinforce a decision to operationalize ADHD in specific ways. Commonly used methodologies also divide those being tested or observed into two (or more) groups, affected or not by ADHD. Statistical methods then often compare the norms of the two groups. In so doing, the research seeks and reinforces differences between "ADHD" and "normal" that solidify the construct used to divide the group in the first place. In these and other ways, scientific methodologies and assumptions shape the ADHD construct, and also stabilize it, making it resistant to change.

Neither of these arguments suggests that ADHD isn't "real." The associated symptoms—subjective and behavioral—the struggles with learning, work, and fitting in, the detectable variations in brain structure and function are all very real. But that does not mean that those real symptoms, signs, and neurological parameters exist with anything like the uniformity accorded to ADHD as defined in the DSM. To claim that ADHD is as distinctive and identifiable as diabetes—to again refer to the American Psychiatric Association's example—is to *reify* it. In contrast, most experts acknowledge that ADHD's presentation is variable, that the boundaries of the diagnosis are fuzzy, and that it is not yet clear what the underlying neurophysiology/ies of ADHD are. But by downplaying that variability in favor of a categorical and reified diagnosis, the experts (along with most of the rest of us) put in place a reified concept—one that has gained multiple facets that do not benefit diagnosable individuals.

Medicine and science, though, are not the only contributors to the present understanding of ADHD. Certainly the pharmaceutical industry has fostered a particular view, in which ADHD is "...an extraordinarily morbid condition...potentially devastating...[with] a very ominous prognosis' (Anonymous, 2005, 12)," urgently requiring treatment with medication to salvage productivity and friendships. But Chapter 3 will demonstrate ways in which the pharmaceutical industry is just one of many social contributors to the concept. The medical world defines mental disorders as impairments relative to socially defined goals and achievements, such as particular ways of interacting with others (not interrupting, not listening when spoken to), kinds of work accomplished, and how the work is accomplished (staying on task, attention to details). Other symptoms are more subjective but still relative to work or school expectations (internal feelings of restlessness during class or meetings). The set of norms ADHD-diagnosable individuals have difficulty in achieving, then, are to a great extent set by social expectations in homes, schools, and the workplace; symptoms observable in each are among the diagnostic criteria. Additionally, social aspects of medicine play a role in characterizing ADHD. Doctors' area of expertise, and their institutional support, is in care of individuals. Unable to intervene with social expectations—although these are, in principle, malleable—clinicians endorse a concept in which the dysfunction is in the individual. Economic considerations pertain as well; clinics and insurance companies need categories, pharmacies need prescriptions. Science, too, participates in socially crafting the diagnosis, by guiding research questions to the framework of "ADHD" to garner funding. Chapter 3 describes these mutual influences as an interaction of a network of allies, drawing on Bruno Latour's actor-network theory.

The choices of the "allies" who have helped structure ADHD might alone be enough to establish that the current understanding of ADHD is to some extent optional. Open questions and critique make the aspect of choice even clearer. There is no tidy match between problems attributed to ADHD and diagnosis and treatment that solves those problems. Although certain treatment successes are common, ADHD diagnosis and treatment do not uniformly solve the problems the category was designed to address, such as impaired (to use the DSM-IV's term) social or organizational skills. Parents and ADHD-diagnosable individuals may also have misgivings about diagnosis and treatment, given overt drug side effects or subtler effects on self-understanding. In addition, both proponents and opponents of the current diagnosis raise concerns over equity in the distribution of diagnosis, treatment, and accommodations by social class, race, and gender—proponents typically argue that not enough is done for a certain group; opponents claim that it's too much.

People who want science to arbitrate such disagreements might protest that our choices about understanding and managing ADHD are not extensive. Of course, they might argue, our concept of ADHD is somewhat shaped by needs, but now and increasingly in the future, science reveals the facts: How brain structure and function relate to objectively defined dysfunction, how treatment works and under what conditions, and so forth. Chapter 4, however, argues against this perspective, casting doubt on the possibility of reaching scientific conclusions on ADHD that do not also embed our interests. This is *not* because the science is overtly biased (say, by pharmaceutical company dollars). Instead, standard practices of clinical science embed social values in scientific methods and conclusions. One contributing factor is that researchers put more emphasis on certain aspects of ADHD, downplaying others. For example, clinical science has emphasized the biology of ADHD and pharmacological solutions, and devoted fewer resources to studying the roles of education and social structure. The emphasis alone gives the appearance that the biological view of ADHD is the one worth studying. More deeply, the concepts and words used to operationalize and interpret data also contain the values that are embedded in the ADHD concept. This marks much of the scientific literature with value-valenced interpretations of what counts as "dysfunction." Specific methodologies also add values to the construct. By continually finding ways in which "ADHD" differs from "normal" on average, science strengthens the distinction and solidifies the association of negative (undesirable) values with ADHD and positive ones with "normal." In the end, the concept that science develops reflects social and scientific values, despite the belief that the sciences of ADHD present objective truths. It also reinforces the values: The status of science as fact producer lends credence to pre-existing social attitudes toward ADHD, establishing a positive feedback loop that strengthens negative associations with ADHD—and with ADHD-diagnosable people.

Chapter 5 argues that the values embedded in our understanding of ADHD, the subtle or not-so-subtle directiveness of our practices, and the limited options available to ADHD-diagnosable individuals combine to create a climate of intolerance toward ADHD-diagnosable individuals. The current intolerance differs from older forms of stigmatization—those who endorse the ADHD concept no longer see diagnosable people as "naughty" or "slackers." Still, the judgments implied by those terms have not disappeared. Rather, they have been transformed into medical oughts: "You ought to get treated," or "You need to get your child treated." Many readers, even if they have been convinced by the elements of choice evident in our views of ADHD, and even if they recognize that the current concept embeds values, will still find this claim counterintuitive. After all, many swear by the benefits they get from diagnosis and treatment, and few are *forced* into treatment. Chapter 5 does not deny this; if people feel they benefit, they do benefit, at least in a way. Yet diagnosis and treatment have downsides. For example, a commonly cited benefit is that diagnosis and treatment enables treated individuals to meet educational and social expectations. But these expectations may be socially designated and culture bound in problematic ways, and, as people meet the expectations, the goals tend to ratchet up, making the benefit short-lived.

The book's final chapter discusses how, given the open options in each venue, we might retain the benefits of diagnosis and treatment for people who want and need it, while reducing intolerance of all diagnosable people. Moving away from current practices is important: Chapter 6 predicts that the new diagnostic criteria in DSM-5 will increase diagnostic rates, likely spreading intolerance to more people. To push toward new alternatives, I recommend four changes:

1. Use a new decision making strategy, the Pragmatist framework, that requires carefully considering facts *and* values in all decisions and actions relevant to ADHD.
2. Avoid dichotomizing.
3. Study new disease models and forms of intervention.
4. Focus less on changing individuals, more on changing society.

Chapter 6 clarifies these recommendations, providing concrete examples and implementation strategies. Each change would contribute to providing positive alternatives to ADHD-diagnosable people. In addition, because similar patterns reinforce intolerance of millions with other clinical diagnoses, adapting the changes could produce more widespread benefits.

More people than I can thank helped me develop the ideas in *Accidental Intolerance*, depending as it does on the work of scientists, clinicians, teachers, philosophers, and other. But, to honor my greatest debts, I would especially like to thank Helen Longino, Carl Elliott, C. Kenneth Waters, Ron Giere, Naomi Scheman, and Valerie Tiberius. Friendly critics at multiple conferences and reading groups improved my focus, and anonymous reviewers of earlier articles and of this book helped me sharpen and clarify the arguments. Readers at various stages helped push it into final form, especially Sam Mitchell, John Sadler, Kristen Intemann, Ramona Ilea, and Katie Plaisance. Students at the University of Minnesota and Mount Holyoke College also offered significant challenges and insights. ADHD professionals in many fields and many ADHD-diagnosed contacts enriched my perspectives. I thank especially Lionel Blatchley, Matthew Burns, Canan Karatekin, Robert Krueger, Monica Luciana, and Tonya White. University of Minnesota research librarians Laurel Haycock and Lisa McGuire, statistician Aaron Rendahl, and Peter Hawthorne assisted with bibliographic research for Chapter 4. Early work on the project was supported by the Mark and Judy Yudof Fellowship and by a Doctoral Dissertation Fellowship from the University of Minnesota. My entire family supported me through my years of work on this project—a special thanks to Lucy for inspiration. Finally, thanks to my canine writing companion Theo, still snoozing at my feet.

REFERENCES

American Psychiatric Association (1994). *Diagnostic and Statistical Manual of Mental Disorders: DSM-IV*, 4 ed. Washington, DC: American Psychiatric Association.

American Psychiatric Association (2000). *Diagnostic and Statistical Manual of Mental Disorders* (4, Text Revision ed.). Arlington, VA: American Psychiatric Association.

American Psychiatric Association (2013). *Diagnostic and Statistical Manual of Mental Disorders: DSM-5* (5th ed.). Washington, DC: American Psychiatric Association.

Anonymous (2005). *Medical Crossfire: Special Edition: Assessing the Safety of ADHD Medications: An Expert Panel Considers the Clinical Significance of Potential Adverse Effects*. (Vol. 6, pp. 1–21). New Brunswick, NJ: University of Medicine and Dentistry of New Jersey and Liberty Communications Network.

Anonymous (2007). AACAP introduces new ADHD practice parameter and pocketcard Retrieved April 29, 2008, from http://www.aacap.org/cs/2007 press releases/aacap_introduces_new_adhd_practice_parameter_and_pocketcard

Barkley, R. A. (1997). *ADHD and the Nature of Self-Control*. New York: The Guilford Press.

Centers for Disease Control and Prevention (2012). 2011–2012 National Survey of Children's Health. Retrieved April 12, 2013, fromhttp://www.cdc.gov/nchs/slaits/nsch.htm.

Clarke, A. R., Barry, R. J., McCarthy, R., Selikowitz, M., & Johnstone, S. J. (2007). Effects of stimulant medications on the EEG of girls with attention-deficit/hyperactivity disorder. *Clinical Neurophysiology, 118,* 2700–2708.

Conrad, P., & Potter, D. (2000). From hyperactive child to ADHD adults: Observatins on the expansion of medical categories. *Social Problems, 47*(4), 559–582.

Faraone, S. V., & Wilens, T. (2003). Does stimulant treatment lead to substance use disorders? *J Clin Psychiatry, 64* (Suppl 11), 9–13.

Hechtman, L., Abikoff, H. B., Klein, R. G., Weiss, G., Respitz, C., Kouri, J., et al. (2004). Academic achievement and emotional status of children with ADHD treated with long-term methylphenidate and multimodal psychosocial treatment. *Journal of the American Academy of Child and Adolescent Psychiatry, 43*(7), 812–819.

Kessler, R. C., Adler, L., Barkley, R., Biederman, J., Conners, C. K., Demler, O., et al. (2006). The prevalence and correlates of adult ADHD in the United States: Results from the National Comorbidity Survey replication. *American Journal of Psychiatry, 163*(4), 716–723.

Zoler, M. L. (2010). Prevalence of ADHD in U.S. youths reached 9.5% in 2007–2008. *Internal Medicine News Digital Network.* Retrieved April 15, 2013, from http://www.internalmedicinenews.com/index.php?id=495&cHash=071010&tx_ttnews[tt_news]=18359

NOTES

1. The DSM-5 (American Psychiatric Association, 2013), was published while *Accidental Intolerance* was in final editing stages. For a discussion of key changes, *see* Chapter 6.
2. Most of the material drawn on in *Accidental Intolerance* was developed during the period the DSM-IV and DSM-IV-TR criteria were in use.

1 ADHD IN MEDICINE

ADHD initiates millions of patient–physician contacts, prescriptions, and referrals every year in the United States. For children and teens, it is the most commonly diagnosed mental disorder. Although many sources, including the American Psychiatric Association's catalog of mental illnesses, the *Diagnostic and Statistical Manual of Mental Disorders* (DSM) (American Psychiatric Association, 2013), estimate that 5% of children and adolescents have ADHD, others suggest higher rates of 8% to 10% (Biederman & Faraone, 2005). Recent practice concurs with the latter: as of 2008, about 9.5% of U. S. children and adolescents had been diagnosed (Froehlich et al., 2007; Merikangas et al., 2010; Centers for Disease Control and Prevention, 2005; Zoler, 2010); by 2011-12, the figure was 11% (Centers for Disease Control and Prevention 2012). Increasingly, too, ADHD is considered a lifelong disorder, beginning in toddlerhood and persisting into adulthood in approximately half of patients.

Medical concepts and practices surrounding ADHD are relatively standardized. Referrals from teachers, questions from parents, or self-identification by adolescents and adults, followed by medical diagnosis and treatment, have become ubiquitous and seemingly natural. But the relatively uniform and routine nature of diagnosis and treatment of ADHD obscures many choices and assumptions underlying current concepts and practices. For each point in the predominant medical view (and its related practices), cogent counterpoints are available. Where the medical view says "biological," a counterpoint says "social"; where medicine says "dysfunction," an alternative view suggests "difference"; where standard views say "categorical," critics say "dimensional."

This chapter aims to clarify rationales for these and other cornerstones of the predominant view and its various alternatives. The first part of this chapter, then, introduces the predominant medical model of ADHD, detailing features that remain controversial, and the second part examines these features to explain the basics of each controversy. Although we will see that some of the current disagreement about ADHD is largely empirical—that is, additional research may readily resolve the issue—other debates are more centrally about differences in values.[1] Opening up a range of alternatives is an important first step in exploring the complexities of the disagreements, and the intermingled roles of facts and values in ADHD concepts and controversies.

Medical Concepts of ADHD

Clinicians aim to help people get well, or to help them manage chronic illness. These practices reflect an underlying commitment to the values of medical practice. Bioethicists capsulize these values in various ways, such as the familiar principles of Beauchamp and Childress (autonomy, beneficence, nonmaleficence, and justice) (Beauchamp & Childress, 2001), or restatements in any number of theoretical terms—utilitarian, feminist, liberal, or religious, among others. In practice, most theories seem at least to emphasize compassion for those who are ill and commitment to delivering care and developing the skills to do so. Compassion for those impaired by ADHD, and commitment to their care, is no exception.

Disease categories are central to this work—differentiating among a cold, strep throat, bronchitis, and pneumonia leads the doctor to different care recommendations for different patients; similarly, differentiating among ADHD, learning disabilities, oppositional defiant disorder, and anxiety disorders leads to different recommendations for different patients. For this reason, how a disease or disorder is *managed* in medicine (the medical practices of diagnosis, treatment, and referral) and how it is *understood* in medicine (the medical concept of a disease category) closely connect. But to see the mutual influences of practices and concepts, it is helpful to consider the two separately.

The Concept, Briefly

ADHD is among the mental disorders listed in the DSM, and the predominant medical view of ADHD accepts the DSM standards as the basis for management decisions. According to the DSM-IV definition, ADHD is a mental disorder in which affected individuals have symptoms or exhibit behaviors of hyperactivity/impulsivity, inattentiveness, or both (*see* Table I.1, Introduction).[2] Three types of ADHD correspond to these possibilities—there is a hyperactive/impulsive type, an inattentive type, and a combined type. Diagnosis requires a cluster of symptoms: an ADHD-diagnosable person must have six of nine symptoms of hyperactivity/impulsivity, six of nine symptoms of inattention, or both. For example, a child with hyperactive/impulsive-type ADHD might fidget excessively in the classroom, frequently blurt out answers, or regularly interrupt others; an adult might feel an internalized restlessness, frequently make "inappropriate" comments, or abuse drugs or alcohol. Individuals of any age with inattentive-type ADHD might daydream or have trouble concentrating on tedious tasks. The symptoms aren't trivial: Diagnosis requires that they impair the individual's function in more than one environment, such as home, school, or work. A large majority of those affected have comorbid diagnoses (coexisting disorders), such as learning disorders, oppositional defiant disorder, conduct disorder, anxiety, or depression (Mayes, Calhoun, & Crowell, 2000; McCracken, 2000). ADHD diagnosis also correlates with long-term difficulties in life experience—for example, relative to non-diagnosable individuals, ADHD-diagnosable people complete fewer years of school, and they have increased risk of accidental injury and higher rates of substance abuse (Biederman et al., 2006; National Institutes of Health, 1998).

The initial cause(s) of ADHD and the mechanism(s) that sustain it are not yet understood. One hypothesis is that dopamine transmission is slowed in ADHD, so that areas of the brain dependent on dopamine for typical function are adversely affected. The most common form of treatment, stimulant medication such as Ritalin or Adderall, is believed to compensate for this underlying dysfunction in dopaminergic pathways, but not to correct that dysfunction permanently. However, norepinephrine or other neurotransmitters may be involved (Tripp & Wickens, 2009). Some studies suggest that variation or delay in brain development is primary (Shaw et al., 2007), and exposure to potential environmental triggers such as maternal smoking during pregnancy, pesticides, television viewing, or lead may predispose children to symptoms (Bouchard, Bellinger, Wright, & Weisskopf, 2010; Froehlich et al., 2009; Linnet et al., 2005; Nigg, Nikolas, Knottnerus, Cavanagh, & Friderici, 2010; Swing, Gentile, Anderson, & Walsh, 2010). ADHD tends to cluster in families (Castellanos & Tannock, 2002), but, as with most complex traits, there is not an obvious single gene or deterministic pattern of heritability (Franke, Neale, & Faraone, 2009; Langley et al., 2004; Ogdie et al., 2003).

Practice

Although classified among the mental disorders, ADHD is most commonly diagnosed and treated by primary care physicians—family physicians, pediatricians, or internists—rather than by psychiatrists. Primary care physicians treat two-thirds to three-quarters of patients, while 12% to 21% are cared for by psychiatrists, and an additional 10% by other specialists (Peterson, Shulman, & Ireys, 2007; Zarin, Tanielian, Suarez, & Marcus, 1998). For many physicians, ADHD represents a significant portion of their patient load. Even in the late 1990s, before the increases in diagnostic rates in the '00s, 3.6% of physician office visits for children aged 5 to 14 years involved ADHD (Zito et al., 1999), as did approximately 1.85% of visits for those under 18 years—more than 3 million visits per year.[3] Subsequently, between 2002 and 2010, prescribed use of ADHD medication by youths increased 46% (Chai et al., 2012), on top of continued growth in the intervening years (Anonymous, 2006); presumably, office visits increased concomitantly.

Usually, someone other than a physician is the first to suggest that a person might have ADHD. According to a survey of physicians in several specialties, school personnel and parents lead 52% and 30% of the time, respectively, whereas physicians are first in about 14% of cases (Sax & Kautz, 2003).[4] Adults typically self-refer—that is, they go to a physician with the suspicion that they might have ADHD. In any case, once the possibility is considered, diagnosis relies heavily on self-report (in the case of adults), or teacher and parent reports in the case of children. However, ruling out situational problems—for example, temporary reactions to stress—is important, as is recognizing coexisting or alternative diagnoses. Specially designed questionnaires such as the Kiddie Schedule for Affective Disorders and Schizophrenia (K-SADS) and the Brown Attention-Deficit Disorder Rating Scale serve to begin this process. Sometimes tests of attention can be useful, but in general with ADHD (as with all mental disorders at present) there are no definitive physiological or psychological tests for the diagnosis. For this reason, the clinician's training and clinical judgment—and the training and judgment of the teacher whose observations are frequently a crucial aspect of the diagnosis—are key determinants of who receives the diagnosis.

Although not all physicians follow the typical pattern, U. S. treatment recommendations are fairly standardized. For example, the treatment parameters adopted by pediatricians and psychiatrists both recommend a trial of non-drug treatment, but early use of stimulant medication as necessary (American Academy of Child and Adolescent Psychiatry, 2002; American Academy of Pediatrics, 2001; Pliszka et al., 2007), providing limited emphasis on or information about other interventions. In practice, this means that a very high percentage of those diagnosed at least make a trial of stimulant medication—for example, between 1991 and 2000, roughly 90% of those receiving an ADHD diagnosis received a prescription for a stimulant (Mayes, Bagwell, & Erkulwater, 2009). Drugs other than stimulants are also sometimes used, and clinicians may also recommend behavioral treatments, specialized educational strategies, and/or accommodations in a diagnosed individual's environment. Not enough is known about environmental precursors of ADHD for clinicians to make specific preventive recommendations, but several practices recommended to parents by the American Academy of Pediatrics and the American College of Obstetrics and Gynecology address potential triggers, among them avoiding smoking during pregnancy, limiting young children's TV viewing, and emphasizing organic foods.

Medical practice suggests focus on particular aspects of ADHD. First, the emphasis on pharmacotherapy reflects physicians' primarily biological interpretation of ADHD symptomatology. In the biological perspective, ADHD is conceived as a biological dysfunction in an individual, involving genetic influences, neurochemistry, or neuroanatomy. A biological perspective does not exclude the roles of society and relationships—even in a disease with well-demarcated biological causes and consequences (an infection, say) social circumstances can contribute to a patient's distress, and an individual's illness can affect behavior and thereby affect others. It does, however, de-emphasize society and relationships in making the biological dysfunction the underlying cause of the patient's impairment or distress and the chief point of intervention.

Second, the aspects of practice that focus on biology relate closely to medical focus on individuals. Although physicians often attend to family units and to how the ADHD-diagnosed individual relates to others, the center of intervention is the diagnosed individual and not the social or familial circumstances. This aspect of practice fits not only with the biological model but also with standards of individualized patient–physician interaction more generally.

Third, physicians rely on a standard diagnosis and (relatively) consistent diagnostic procedures because their ability to intervene effectively depends on their identifying ADHD as correctly as possible. Identifiability, like the individual and biological focus, is central to practice.

Fourth, the care is also a complex economic exchange, involving physician, patient, insurance companies, government, the pharmaceutical industry, and various other professionals and employees. The scope of these exchanges is large: healthcare expenses for ADHD-diagnosable individuals have been "conservatively estimated" at $3.3 billion each year (Centers for Disease Control and Prevention, 2005, 847). United States sales of medication alone have been estimated at $2.3 billion,[5] and a typical diagnostic work-up for ADHD costs $2,000 (Diller, 2006).

Along with the commitment to medical values, the foci on biology, individuals, identifiability, and economic exchange that characterize practice shape the concept of ADHD in complex ways.

The Concept, Detail

The predominant medical concept of ADHD nests within several "layers." Most general are concepts of disease, physical and mental; second are general understandings of mental illness or disorder; third, the particular definition of "mental disorder" adopted in the DSM; and fourth, the criteria that specify the constellation of symptoms termed "ADHD." These, in turn, interact with the broad set of practices and values that frame the practice of medicine, eventually culminating, for clinicians and their patients, in the specificities of the individual consultation and recommendations. Controversies rooted in each level persist in debates over ADHD.

Disease

Disease definitions can be surprisingly difficult to pin down. Diseases are not simply uncomfortable or painful conditions—some, like hypertension (high blood pressure) or hypercholesterolemia (high cholesterol), are not. One might think that diseases are relatively uncommon, compared with "normal" states, but that would not be true of dental caries (cavities) or, increasingly, obesity. Nor do diseases necessarily decrease reproductive fitness or shorten life—for example, Parkinson's disease does neither. Disruption, maldevelopment, or misdirection—in short, dysfunction—of some aspect of an individual's typical biological status seems nearly universal, until one recognizes that the line between function and dysfunction is indistinct (where does one draw the lines to mark high blood pressure, high cholesterol, obesity?) and that not all diseases involve dysfunctions (for example, although infectious diseases disrupt function, the body's responses to invasion are arguably functional). Most diseases seem to be properties of individuals, but others are dysfunctions only relative to contingent social factors (some disabilities dissipate with environmental changes). Correspondingly, philosophers of medicine, as well as physicians, have debated disease definitions that emphasize these and other criteria. Many of the criteria are particularly problematic in the context of mental disease (or disorder) definitions, owing to the complexity of mental capacities, the relatively poorly understood biological basis of mental functions, and the prominent social and relational factors in many mental disorders.

Brief History of "Mental Disorder"

The designation "mental disorder," or its historical cognates, serves in part to explain aberrant and undesired behavior and in part to ground differential treatment of those judged to be mentally disordered—for example, to legitimize medication or institutionalization. Historically, primarily physiological explanations, such as Galenic theories of imbalanced bodily humors, have alternated with psychological or spiritual notions, centering on stresses and anxieties, or on demonic possession. The changing concepts shifted management practices as well, which at various times emphasized the physical, the punitive, the spiritual, or the protective, in practices of (for example) blood letting, imprisonment, exorcism, or humane isolation.

Competition between physiological and psychological emphases, and their respective management strategies, carried into the twentieth and twenty-first centuries. In the past hundred years, Western psychiatrists and psychologists introduced a succession of concepts to explain mental function and dysfunction: psychodynamic, behaviorist, humanist, cognitive, neuroscientific, and other systems competed. In the early 1900s, psychological theories predominated. Psychodynamic models of mental disorder, for example, conceived the symptoms as conflicts between levels of function that were not distinctly different from normal in cause or kind (Reznek, 1991). Clinicians were oriented toward the individual and toward complexity, rather than toward diagnosis of discrete disease entities. In mid-century, behaviorists emphasized the environment–person interaction in their theorizing; they suggested that mental disorders, like other behaviors, were learned responses.

Meanwhile, however, scientists in other disciplines studied neuroanatomy, neurophysiology, and, eventually, the biochemistry and genetics of mental illness. Increasing knowledge in these areas, along with advances in pharmaceutical treatment of mental disorders, helped reorient psychiatrists' allegiances and concepts of mental disorder toward physiological theories. As psychiatry aligned itself more closely with medicine in the 1970s (psychology, from which psychiatry grew, was historically a branch of philosophy), it incorporated the various mental perturbations that dynamic psychiatrists and psychoanalysts had treated into the DSM disease categories (Horwitz, 2002). At the same time, the division between psychiatry and psychology in the study of abnormal and normal mental processes and behaviors, respectively, remained largely intact (not completely so, as those in the subfields of abnormal and clinical psychology, among others, would object). Thus, in the United States, physiological theories, the field of psychiatry, and the DSM nosology now predominate in the study and treatment of mental disorders, but many other theories, disciplines, and several alternative nosologies compete.

A crucial aspect of this evolution is that in the early twentieth century, psychiatrists began treating not just the small class of people who were severely mentally impaired but also those with less catastrophically disabling conditions, such as neuroses, addictions, and problems in living (Horwitz, 2002; Lunbeck, 1994). More recently, a National Comorbidity Survey found that by today's standards, 46% of people suffer from a mental disorder at some point in life (Kessler et al., 2005); ADHD is one of the most common.

Mental Disorder

Different models of mental disorder emphasize biology, sociality, cognition, and human distress to varying degrees. Biological models—the most common for ADHD—emphasize biological dysfunction. Psychodynamic models emphasize relations, as well as mental processing of those relations. Stress-diathesis and biopsychosocial models attempt to balance complex interactions among contributing factors. Debates about the different models are not idle academic exercises. Different models yield different nosologies (classes of mental disorder), varying hypotheses about causes of disease or distress, and different types of treatment; they also encourage different attitudes toward those who have mental disorders.

Two aspects of the debates over concepts of mental disorder are particularly important with respect to understanding the status of ADHD. First, it is not clear how to interpret, or how much to emphasize, the "levels" involved in the phenomenology of mental illness. Roughly, mental disorders involve biological, psychological, and social levels—but these, too, can be subdivided. "Biology" works at the levels of the entire body (brain, the rest of the body, neural and hormonal directions), as well as at molecular, neuronal, and neural pathway levels; "psychology" is both conscious and unconscious and richly complex in each area; and social levels range from close interpersonal relationships to complex institutional and government structures. All of these, it turns out, are relevant to ADHD, and their precise relations to one another and their effects on one another are, at present, unclear.

Second, although most levels can be investigated with empirical techniques (some psychological phenomena still escape this possibility), another "level" also may also affect our interpretation of our observations—the level of *values*. For example, as with physical parameters, what psychological capacities are appropriately called "functions" as opposed to "dysfunctions" can be problematic. Is the demarcation simply a matter of determining statistical norms? Or does it, instead, involve considering what capacities are useful (so we like them) or not useful (so we don't), or which please rather than frustrate or distress us? We need to determine how what we value pertains to what we term a mental disorder and to what we term ADHD in particular.

Debates over mental disorder concepts focus to a great extent on these two issues—the relations among the "levels" and the degree to which the concepts are value-laden. In the case of ADHD, these issues play out complexly— indeed, the debates will be evident throughout the succeeding chapters—and different practitioners hold different views of the appropriate way to understand ADHD. Nevertheless, there is a predominant model of ADHD: the medical model.

A Medical Model of Mental Disorder

What then, are mental disorders, according to a standard medical model? Like other models of mental disorder, medical models pick out conditions *related to higher mental functions*—that is, not to "lower" brain activities like regulation of breathing, heart rate and hormonal systems but to "higher" functions like cognition, attention, and regulation of emotions. A medical model (Institute of Medicine, 1992; Reznek, 1991) conceives medically legitimate mental disorders—those the medical community accepts—as:

- Biological
- Dysfunctions, that are
- Features of individuals
- Identifiable
- Causally explicable via scientific methods (at least in principle), and
- Amenable to medical treatment (at least in principle)

Each of these parallels features of current medical practice, with its emphasis on biology, individuals, identifiability, and economic exchange. The emphasis on pharmacotherapy parallels the biological concept; in the case of mental disorders, the primary (but not sole or necessary) locus of biological dysfunction is the brain. The designation "dysfunction" is often, but not always, tied to the distress of the diagnosable individual. In some cases, the diagnosable individual is not aware of impairment—instead, others notice it. Sociopathic individuals, for example, do not recognize the distress they cause others in their pursuit of their own goals; and children who have symptoms of hyperactivity may not be at all disturbed by their own behavior, but those around them commonly are. In any case, dysfunction gives the rationale for treatment, and the individual is the focus of that treatment and the clinical interaction. Identifiability per se is important—the physician needs parameters for diagnosis, including a diagnostic category. The fifth and sixth criteria are qualified as "in principle" because before these criteria are met there is often a stage in which researchers note that a set of signs and/or symptoms cluster (form a "syndrome"), but for which they cannot yet provide a unifying causal explanation that would facilitate physiological testing and targeted treatment. The criteria also help form the foundation for the economic exchange. ADHD is, of course, among the accepted categories.

DSM Model of Mental Disorders

The DSM

The DSM nosology (a nosology is a classification of diseases) is the de facto guide to what counts as mental disorder in the United States. Not surprisingly, given that psychiatry is a branch of medicine, the DSM model of mental disorder is for the most part consistent with the medical model described above.[6] But examining the DSM definition in more detail is important not only because of the DSM's prominence but also because some debates concerning ADHD relate specifically to the DSM model. The DSM-IV's introduction defines mental disorder as:

> In DSM-IV, each of the mental disorders is conceptualized as a clinically significant behavioral or psychological syndrome or pattern that occurs in an individual and that is associated with present distress (e.g., a painful symptom) or disability (i.e., impairment in one or more important areas of functioning) or with a significantly increased risk of suffering death, pain, disability, or an important loss of freedom. In addition, this syndrome or pattern must not be merely an expectable and culturally sanctioned response to a particular event, for example, the death of a loved one. Whatever its original cause, it must currently be considered a manifestation of behavioral, psychological, or biological dysfunction in the individual. Neither deviant behavior (e.g., political, religious, or sexual) nor conflicts that are primarily between the individual and society are mental disorders unless the deviance or conflict is a symptom of a dysfunction in the individual, as described above (American Psychiatric Association, 2000, xxxi).

The DSM model accords with the medical model in that it emphasizes that a mental disorder is a "dysfunction" and that the dysfunction is "in the individual." Like the medical model, the DSM does not require that the diagnosable individual be aware of distress; this allows treatment of conditions that are observed to be disabling mainly by people other than the patient, such as ADHD in a young child. However, the observed pattern cannot be a culturally typical response to circumstance, nor can it be overtly politically motivated. Finally, the disorder must be "clinically significant"—that is, it needs to be impairing enough (in the judgment of the clinician) that it requires treatment recommended, prescribed, or carried out by a clinician.

A prominent feature of DSM-IV and -5 categories is that each mental disorder is conceived *categorically*. That is, the mental disorders are not conceived as gradients along a continuum (for example, from hypoactive to typically active to hyperactive), as they would be in a *dimensional* system, but rather as having a distinct cutoff point denoting illness. The cutoff points are based not on a single symptom but on an individual having a certain number of symptoms from a list, which details behaviors or symptoms that can be observed by an individual or his/her contacts and/or experienced by the individual. Someone who has fewer symptoms from the lists does not have a less severe form of the disorder; rather, s/he does not have the disorder. Each behavior or symptom considered individually is outside of statistical norms for frequency of occurrence, type, adaptation to circumstances, or other criterion. For example, with ADHD symptoms, one DSM-IV criterion is "often easily distracted by extraneous stimuli." The qualification "often" differentiates the diagnosable individual's experience of inattention from the otherwise nearly universal experience of occasional distractibility. The behaviors or symptoms in the lists have been shown to cluster (that is, to appear together in various combinations)—hence, the content of the lists. For a diagnosis of ADHD, the patient must have six or more symptoms or behaviors from the list for inattention, six from the list for hyperactivity/impulsivity, or both.[7] Clinicians do not use the model rigidly: Clinical medicine is devoted to the care of individuals, and clinicians frequently make exceptions as needed in clinical care. But the categorical model does fit well with certain aspects of practice—determining who should receive treatment, referrals, and billing and insurance claims.

A notable difference between the DSM-IV and medical models is that the medical model specifies that a mental disorder should have a biological cause, while the DSM leaves the door open to behavioral or psychological causes of symptoms as well. However, present-day psychiatrists typically adopt the explicitly biological perspective characteristic of a medical model. For example, a recent study assessed implicit models of mental disorder used by mental health professionals in various fields (Colombo, Bendelow, Fulford, & Williams, 2003; Fulford & Colombo, 2004). Ninety-one percent of the psychiatrists responded to a case history in a way consistent with a medical model, despite their saying they employed a biopsychosocial model in practice. The responses of psychiatric nurses and social workers were more varied.[8] The psychiatrists' responses concur with the emphasis on medication in ADHD treatment, and also with the practice of other physicians. In short, despite the DSM's open door, a medical model of ADHD predominates. The concept is consistent with the DSM model of mental disorder, and shaped by the DSM's categorical criterion and its disorder-specific symptomatology.

ADHD Category

ADHD was conceptualized in close to its modern form in 1980, with the publication of DSM-III, but it has earlier precursors. What follows is a mere sketch of the history; others have recently traced ADHD's historical precursors more completely (Mayes et al., 2009; Rafalovich, 2004).

Brief History

In the early twentieth century, clinicians observed a pattern of hyperactivity and poor attention span in children who recovered from encephalitis, an inflammation of the brain caused by a virus. By the 1960s, researchers identified children with similar symptoms (impulsivity had been added) but no recognized prior illness. The second edition of the *Diagnostic and Statistical Manual of Mental Disorders* (DSM-II), published in 1968, classified this syndrome as "Hyperkinetic reaction of childhood (or adolescence)," placing it among the "Behavior Disorders of Childhood and Adolescence." The syndrome was understood to be "more stable, internalized, and resistant to treatment than *Transient situational disturbances* (q.v.) but less so than *Psychoses, Neuroses,* and *Personality disorders* (q.v.) (American Psychiatric Association, 1968, 50)." The complete diagnostic criteria for hyperkinetic reaction were:

> This disorder is characterized by overactivity, restlessness, distractibility, and short attention span, especially in young children; the behavior usually diminishes in adolescence. (American Psychiatric Association, 1968, 50)

This was followed by one sentence concerning differential diagnosis: "If this behavior is caused by organic brain damage, it should be diagnosed under the appropriate non-psychotic *organic brain syndrome* (q.v.) (American Psychiatric Association, 1968, 50)." Excluding organic brain damage and using the term "reaction" indicate that this ADHD-like disorder was understood on a psychodynamic model (Eisenberg, 1972). Nevertheless, children with this diagnosis were increasingly treated with the stimulants methylphenidate (Ritalin), which was introduced in 1955, or dextroamphetamine: By 1970 an estimated 150,000 to 200,000 children were being treated in the United States, with numbers expected to rise (Grinspoon & Singer, 1973). The 1968 criteria do not list specific behaviors or particular environments in which the characteristic types of behavior occur. But by the early 1970s, focus on behavior in school is obvious in both clinical and education literatures. Psychologists and educators designed special classrooms and/or behavior modification therapies to accommodate or counteract children's symptoms (Krauch, 1971; Miller, 1973), and physicians, social workers, and others also contributed to managing hyperkinesis in the schools.[9]

Increased interest in the inattention component of "hyperkinesis" led to renaming and redefining the category as attention-deficit disorder (ADD) in the third edition of the DSM (Baird, Stevenson, & Williams, 2000; American Psychiatric Association, 1980). DSM-III replaced the DSM-II'S psychodynamic model with descriptive lists of symptoms intended to be agnostic about causation, but with a longer-term goal of orienting psychiatry to empirical and physiological approaches compatible with the rest of medicine. The concerns of teachers and parents about school behavior were reflected in the ADD diagnostic criteria, which emphasize classroom-associated symptoms such as "difficulty concentrating on schoolwork (43)" "frequently calls out in class (44)" and "difficulty staying seated (44)." The descriptive preface to the specific criteria also notes home-based problems such as "failure to follow through on parental requests and instructions (41)." The DSM-III separates symptoms into three categories of inattention, impulsivity, and hyperactivity.

The next version of the DSM, DSM-III-R (American Psychiatric Association, 1987), retained this basic approach but refocused the diagnostic category from "Attention Deficit Disorder (with or without hyperactivity)" to "Attention Deficit Hyperactivity Disorder (mild, moderate, or severe)." The DSM-III-R does not group the symptoms according to descriptions like "hyperactivity" or "inattention," instead presenting a single list. It also places more emphasis than DSM-III on problematic behaviors toward peers, and it notes more comorbidities. Another important change is that the descriptive material discusses work situations; DSM-III criteria mention affected adults only once.

Continuing the practice of listing descriptive symptoms, DSM-IV (American Psychiatric Association, 1994) and DSM-IV-TR (American Psychiatric Association, 2000) reverted to divided symptom lists, this time those reflecting inattention and hyperactivity-impulsivity. Statistical analyses of field trial data showed that the symptoms clustered into these two groups and determined the number of symptoms needed from the list for reliable diagnoses (Lahey et al., 1994). Thus, DSM-IV differentiates three types of ADHD: predominantly inattentive, predominantly hyperactive-impulsive, and combined types. As with other mental disorders, the diagnostic criteria specify the behaviors that signal dysfunction; these are behaviors that either interfere with others (teachers, parents, peers) or correlate with milestones or events deemed undesirable for the ADHD-diagnosable individual (for example, with poor reading scores or increased risk of substance abuse). DSM-IV-TR provides greatly expanded detail and examples in the textual description, and the list of comorbidities is expanded again. Each version beyond DSM-II notes the possibility that a child's symptoms are situational: If the behavior is an expected response to an "inadequate, disorganized, or chaotic environment," then the child does not have ADD or ADHD.

Looking to the Future

The DSM-5, published while *Accidental Intolerance* was in proofs, alters but does not overhaul the DSM-IV-TR criteria. Chapter 6 discusses the likely impact.

Alternative Models, Decision Points

ADHD has been much discussed in the popular press as well as in medical and scientific literatures. Controversies about the predominant medical/DSM model are similarly ubiquitous. Some objections to this view are simply ill-informed. Many, though, stem from cogent questioning of assumptions or hypotheses on which the model is based: its biological basis, status as dysfunctional or as a mental disorder, locus in the individual, degree of identifiability, amenability to treatment, categorical definition, relation to specific diagnostic criteria in the DSM definition, and more. The objections form a complex mix in which some criticisms are largely of the empirical base of the diagnosis (that is, of facts), while others primarily criticize values embedded in the concept. The two types of objections do not separate cleanly, nor, I will argue in later chapters, do facts and values separate cleanly in general. As a starting point, though, we can roughly divide the issues into those that are relatively empirical and those that emphasize differences in values. For the former, a need for more research is central to the controversy. These issues are often (though not always) scientific experts' disputes, which are the subject of Chapters 2 and 4. Among them are different hypotheses concerning the etiology of ADHD; the efficacy of treatment protocols; and some aspects of the validity of the characterization of ADHD—including questions about its subdivisions, comorbidities, boundaries, gender differences, and dimensionality. The (primarily) value-based objections may come from ADHD experts, but they also come from interested outsiders—scientists, scholars, physicians, and mental health professionals in related and unrelated fields, teachers and school administrators, parents, affected individuals, and others. Examining a number of these objections will show why the familiar medical model remains contentious, as well as illustrating reasonable alternatives to the model.

Disorder, Dysfunction, and Values

One long-standing dispute in philosophy of medicine is the extent to which concepts of disease are or can be value free. Some argue that the distinction between healthy and diseased states can be drawn without reference to values, others that values are central to this distinction. The debate centers on whether diseases can be understood simply as biological phenomena or whether people's dislike of "disease" makes the notion fundamentally evaluative.

Christopher Boorse argues in favor of a value-free notion of "disease," but this concept is not equivalent to current understandings of mental disorder. "Mental disorder," he says, contains two distinguishable components (Boorse, 1975): a nonevaluative component, mental *disease,* which should be distinguished from the evaluative component, mental *illness.* "Disease," whether mental or physical, is merely a disruption of an internal state or a limitation of function caused by an environmental agent—that is, a biological dysfunction. Its converse, health, is conformity to species design. Similarly, "function" is not an evaluative concept: We do not call a process a "function" because it does something we like. Rather, "a function in the biologist's sense is nothing but a standard causal contribution to a goal actually pursued by the organism (Boorse, 1975, 57)." Mental *illnesses,* in contrast, are understood according to value-valenced norms: They are undesirable for the ill, entitle the affected individual to treatment, and provide an excuse for behaviors (Boorse, 1975; Boorse, 1976). Boorse suggests that, to the extent possible, we limit the categories of mental illnesses by requiring that they also be mental diseases.

At present, few mental disorders meet Boorse's proposed requirement: the empirical evidence for biological dysfunction in most DSM-defined mental disorders, including ADHD, is at best incomplete (more on this in Chapter 2). In addition, although Boorse carves out some areas of the mental disorder concept that are *not* value free (those associated with mental illness), his argument that the concept of mental disease *is* value free depends on his argument that biological function and dysfunction are value-free concepts—but several theorists have argued that they are not. A very straightforward argument is that "functions" simply are valued operations or mechanisms,[10] "dysfunctions" the opposite (Megone, 2000). Similar reasoning applies to Boorse's teleological definition of functions in terms of "goals." Even in the case of animal or plant diseases, the conclusion that a variation is dysfunctional requires a value judgment pegged to goals imputed to the organism, such as survival.

Another point used against Boorse's view (and those of Wakefield and Schwartz, which will be discussed shortly) is that (biological) dysfunction alone cannot demarcate mental disease. Instead, dysfunction must be defined relative to an environment—what is dysfunctional in one set of circumstances may be functional in another (Murphy & Woolfolk, 2001). For example, ADHD-associated traits might have been beneficial in some environments, explaining why they are common today despite no longer being useful (Grady et al., 2003; Murphy & Woolfolk, 2001). More generally, determining which traits are functional and which dysfunctional requires taking into account the environment, as well as evaluative criteria that assess benefit or harm.

Wakefield takes another tack. With his "harmful dysfunction analysis" of mental disorder, he posits that harm and dysfunction are both necessary elements of the single concept. In his words, "attribution of disorder requires not only a scientific judgment that a condition is due to an internal dysfunction, but also a value judgment that the condition in question is harmful to the individual or to society (Wakefield, 2002, 148)." According to Wakefield, a scientific judgment of dysfunction is apt—and value free—when a biologically designed function fails to perform as it was designed to do during its evolution. To the extent that mental disorders are attributable to such functional failures, they are neither value valenced nor culturally relative. However, in Wakefield's view, values entailed by the notion of "harm" *must* contribute to attributions of disorder. Not only does this capture present usage, in Wakefield's view, but requiring the value component has heuristic benefits: It encourages a close look at what *sorts* of harm are intended by attributions of mental disorder. These amendments better capture the current understanding of mental disorder, in that the concept is not divided as Boorse suggests. Still, Wakefield's view that the scientific judgment of dysfunction is value free is subject to the same objections that counter Boorse's view.[11]

Fulford points out that the value-ladenness of disease concepts applies to physical as well as mental disorders—it is just less apparent that values are in play when the disorder in question is physical (Fulford, 2004). This is because disvaluation of outcomes typical of physical disorders, such as pain and death, is nearly universal—making the involved values function like facts—while people have valid disagreements about what constitutes harm stemming from atypical mental capacities and behaviors. Similarly, normal function is understood more uniformly for physical than for mental functions—mechanisms that contribute to physical survival are very widely agreed to be functions, but for mental mechanisms, modes and degrees of flourishing are various enough that agreement is not as complete.

In my view, "dysfunction," "disease," and "mental disorder" are all inescapably evaluative concepts—but my reasons for thinking so will not be clear until Chapter 4, where I show how values influence scientific concepts. In any case, disagreements over what constitutes harm, dysfunction, or impairment form the basis of much friction concerning ADHD: ADHD experts and non-experts disagree over whether ADHD-associated traits and behaviors should be considered dysfunctional at all, and they differ over the frequency or severity of symptoms that should be considered dysfunctional. Ongoing controversies concerning overdiagnosis of ADHD (too much behavior or symptoms classified as dysfunctional) or underdiagnosis (too little) centers on such disagreements. Similarly, alternative models of mental disorder generally, and of ADHD in particular, embed values that differ from those in the medical/DSM model. Such disagreements reveal ways in which the categories we use to describe mental disorders are flexible, embedding options based on different interpretations of facts, using a variety of values.

Line Drawing, Dysfunction, and Difference

Although not all theorists agree, choices about "line drawing" demonstrate that "disease" and "disorder" are flexible categories, and also represent one way values affect medical models of mental disorder. Many biomedical phenomena fall on a continuum, rather than being either present or absent, "on" or "off," sick or well. Blood pressure, for example, ranges from low to typical to high. Deciding what level separates the disease "hypertension" (high blood pressure) from a high normal reading involves drawing a metaphorical line somewhere along the continuum. Similarly, line drawing is needed to establish cut-off points for ADHD diagnosis. Presently, in ADHD's categorical conception, line drawing establishes the number of symptoms needed for diagnosis. If ADHD turns out, empirically, to be better understood as a dimensional category (or categories), line drawing would be needed to establish the points(s) on relevant continua (for example, the level of activity) that would demarcate disorder.

Schwartz argues that line drawing can be done in a way that eases "worries that drawing a line between functioning and dysfunctioning inevitably relies on problematic teleological assumptions or value judgments (Schwartz, 2007, 384)."[12] His basic approach is to decouple the concept of dysfunction from concerns about the consequences of the dysfunctions. To draw a line correctly on, for example, a bell-curve distribution, such as that of blood pressure, one needs two sets of information: One set is the frequencies in a reference class of measurements associated with the trait or condition (such as systolic and diastolic blood pressure, measured in mmHg, in the class of 55- to 65-year-old males); the other is the "facts about negative consequences" of a trait or condition (Schwartz, 2007, 377). The second set of information provides a rationale for the line-drawing, which otherwise must be done arbitrarily. A common condition with serious negative consequences might be rightly termed a disease in a large portion of a population—again, dental caries is an example. In contrast, a population might vary according to a certain functional trait but have no members with negative consequences despite the variation; in this case the statistical outliers would not be diseased.

Schwartz's account nicely clarifies one way values concerning negative consequences are embedded in the criteria for specific diseases, but in my view, despite his stated goal of tempering the role of values, this clarification does not eliminate values from disease accounts. Saying that the second criterion involves "facts about negative consequences" simply pushes the issue one step back—to determining what counts as "negative" (and as a *fact about* what is negative, though that's another issue). "Negative consequences" exist only with respect to some set of values: in medicine, such determinations are based on judgments of clinical importance. These judgments—value judgments—are needed to interpret data and to draw lines demarcating disease.

Line drawing is an ongoing issue in debates over ADHD. As we have seen, lines as drawn by DSM-IV criteria result in diagnostic rates of approximately 11%. Yet, looking beyond that simple average reveals significantly different results in different cases: Comparing diagnosis rates among the youngest and oldest students within grades shows that the younger students—who are less mature in behavior and intellectual development than their older classmates—have an ADHD diagnosis rate 28% to 60% (Elder, 2010) higher than that of their older classmates (Evans, Morrill, & Parente, 2010) and stimulant use nearly double. Lines drawn by criteria of the similar category, hyperkinesis, in the *International Classification of Disease* (ICD), result in diagnostic rates as low as 1% (Dopfner, Breuer, Wille, Erhart, & Ravens-Sieberer, 2008; World Health Organization, 2002). For these and other reasons, the "correct" diagnostic rate continues to be debatable. Line drawing also exposes the option of *not* drawing a line to distinguish health and disease. An alternative, in cases of dispute, is to instead consider variations in function as *differences* rather than dysfunctions. In the case of a DSM-defined mental disorder like ADHD—one that is often relatively mild and not necessarily experienced as having negative consequences by the diagnosable individual—this approach appears appropriate to some.

Categorical vs. Dimensional Concepts

As we have seen, the DSM's categorical conception is the predominant model of mental disorders generally, and of ADHD in particular. Other models are also in use, however, and it may well be the case that different models are suitable for different mental disorders. Psychologist Nick Haslam argues that, empirically, mental disturbances are of heterogeneous types (Haslam, 2003). Some, such as neuroticism, are "non-kinds": psychological continua or dimensions along which there is *no* principled way to mark a division between health and disease. "Practical kinds" are also dimensional, but pragmatic criteria, such as a need to prescribe treatment, provide a principled way to mark the division. (Suitability of a model is partly empirical, relating to a model's accuracy in describing a disorder and guiding treatment, but the choice typically also has other rationales and important consequences.) Haslam argues that depression is a practical kind. "Fuzzy kinds" are discontinuous to an extent, but the boundary between the fuzzy kind and non-members of the kind is not sharp: Some individuals are clearly members of a fuzzy-kind set such as borderline personality disorder, others are clearly not, and a third group is intermediate or indeterminate. "Discrete kinds" are clearly dichotomous with non-members of the discrete-kind set; Haslam suggests that the severe form of depression termed melancholia may be of this type. "Natural kinds," rare in psychiatry, have a simple and direct relationship to underlying physiology: Biological trait X always results in mental disorder Y; Haslam gives the example of Williams syndrome, a result of a minute chromosome deletion. Only discrete kinds and natural kinds fit empirically with a categorical view of mental disorders. Thus, categorical conceptions are often scientifically inaccurate (Clark, 2005), although they may answer practical needs. In Haslam's view, a nosology that took the different possibilities into account would be better informed, both theoretically and empirically.

In addition to pointing out the scientific inaccuracies of the DSM's categorical model, critics argue that it creates clinical problems (First, 2005; Kupfer, 2005).[13] First, it encourages reducing the line-drawing problem to counting symptoms from a list. This means that alternative rationales for applying (or not applying) a diagnostic category are less likely to be employed, reducing diagnostic sensitivity to individual circumstances. Second, because the symptoms are often not unique to individual diagnoses, categories overlap extensively, complicating diagnosis and treatment. Third, despite the seeming clarity of lists, the symptoms on the lists vary greatly, as do the comorbidities and, presumably, the underlying causes of the symptoms. The result is extensive heterogeneity among people given a single diagnostic label.

One option for change is to adopt a dimensional model of classification which, by employing several dimensions of variation, could individualize a profile of a patient's mental disorder(s) and encourage more specificity in treatment (Widiger & Samuel, 2005, 500). Dimensional classifications could also better represent general vulnerability to overlapping diagnoses, potentially improving both treatment and prevention efforts (Brown & Barlow, 2005). Psychodynamic models are also available: The authors of the *Psychodynamic Diagnostic Manual* (PDM) suggest that more individualized diagnoses and treatment plans are needed (PDM Task Force, 2006). Psychodynamic models also shift the emphasis of symptomatology from objective—symptoms and behaviors that are other-defined and catalogued—to subjective. The subjective view emphasizes the experience of affected individuals, and the complexity of the full range of mental functioning. The shift in perspective, the PDM argues, refocuses on "the whole person," rather than the disorder.

These are general considerations, relevant to a range of mental disorders. What about ADHD in particular? Reasearchers have proposed several dimensional models of ADHD. One approach retains symptom clusters similar to the current groupings but would assess patients on a scale of severity—for example, Neuman et al. (1999) proposed two dimensions, one corresponding to the inattentive symptoms, another including both inattentive and hyperactive/impulsive symptoms.[14] Others have suggested that ADHD might be modeled in multidimensional terms involving Conscientiousness, Neuroticism, and Agreeableness—three of the "Big Five" dimensions of personality (Nigg et al., 2002); assessment would determine where patients fell on each continuum. Haslam et al. (2006) propose that ADHD be modeled along a single-dimension severity scale. Their reasoning is based on their taxometric analysis showing that ADHD has *no* latent structure. The lack of a latent structure suggests that there is no single underlying dysfunction causing the disorder—that is, ADHD is a pragmatic kind.[15] For this reason, they argue, the diagnostic lines must be based not on physiological signs, or on categorical lists, but according to clinical judgment of impairment.

In the near future, these are theoretical debates: The DSM-5 model of ADHD is not dimensional. In part, this is a judgment that the science of ADHD does not yet support any causal model[16]; the DSM criteria set (ostensibly) leaves this open. In large part, though, it is a pragmatic decision. Current needs of practice in medicine, education, and disability services and accommodation for adults require specific diagnostic categories, despite ADHD's known fuzzy boundaries, heterogeneity, and comorbidities.

As in the general case, however, the persistence of categorical models is contentious for the values it embeds and the consequences it encourages. The DSM's categorical diagnoses, in their alignment with the remainder of medicine, are greatly influenced by the pragmatics of care. The relative strictness of the DSM classification, with its objective symptom lists and categorical diagnoses, simplifies diagnosis and treatment by involving fewer individual determinations than a dimensional or psychodynamic model would (First, 2005; Kupfer, 2005). In being thus (in principle) clear cut, categorical diagnoses emphasize reasoned distribution of care, cost-efficacy, and efficiency, paralleling a focus in the rest of medicine on valuing these parameters. The PDM, in contrast, would emphasize complexity, global functioning, and subjective experience, evidencing a worldview that prioritizes interactivity and subjective phenomenology.[17] Some dimensional models would value context and individualization over simplicity, although it is not clear that Haslam's single-dimension model would do so. Again, the various values embedded in the models would affect implementation, directly impacting diagnosis and treatment.

Another crucial impact, which will receive much fuller treatment in subsequent chapters, is that categorical models dichotomize groups: some people have ADHD, others do not. In making this distinction, they create the possibility of negative judgments of the dichotomized group. Dimensional and psychodynamic models, although not fully immune from such results, soften the dichotomization in their explicit recognition that there is no difference in kind among people on the dimension or reaction in question, but only a difference in degree.

Medical(ization) vs. Social

As we saw earlier, it was not long ago that there was no such thing as "ADHD"—no medical category into which people with ADHD-associated traits and behaviors could be placed. Instead, people thought of those diagnosable by today's standards in social or moral terms: depending on comorbidities, the term might be "class clown," "Tom-boy," "day-dreamer," "failure," "juvenile delinquent," or other appellation. Today, ADHD, along with many other mental disorders currently in the DSM, is "medicalized" rather than moralized. Critics think this change has gone too far or has gone astray. Their ideas help display the basic assumptions of the medical model (the biological basis, locus in individuals, amenability to treatment, etc.), the values embedded in those assumptions, and alternatives to them.

One way think about the medical model of mental disorders is to consider its fit with medical practice. Despite a few decades of increasing attention to patient autonomy, it is still the case that physicians determine who fits which diagnostic categories and who (at least among those with means to pay) receives treatment. From the perspective of medical practice, this process exhibits the medical value of compassion for those who suffer, as well as a determination that the suffering is caused by a condition amenable to medical treatment. In acting on this value and judgment, it is also the case that physicians—and the medical system that supports them—exert significant control. Conrad and Schneider (1992 [1980]) describe medicalization as a shift of social control from older forms, such as the church and the legal system, to medicine. They suggest that this trend is positive in its humanitarian emphasis, and in its extension of a nonpunitive, nonblaming "sick role" to distressed people who might previously have been considered morally depraved or legally culpable. On the other hand, they argue, the values reinforced by models of mental disorder and medical practices of diagnosis and treatment are those of the people or institutions who have "the power to legitimate their definitions" (Conrad & Schneider, 1992 [1980], 29). People declared mentally ill may not be blamed, but they are nevertheless judged according to those definition, and they are nevertheless obligated, as part of the sick role, to alter their behavior. A physician's decision that a child's behavior is uncontrollably disruptive for his/her family or classmates is often a significant part of determining that the child has an impairment, has ADHD, and needs medication to manage his/her actions. In adults, the result is the "medicalization of underperformance" (Conrad & Potter, 2000, 573).

Thinking of ADHD as (at least in part) a disorder of social expectations draws attention to the details of those expectations as embedded in ADHD criteria. The diagnostic criteria, by defining symptoms as departures from certain norms, place value on certain forms of school and work achievement, orderliness, focus, persistence, carefulness, attentiveness, attention to detail, and defined social behaviors such as not interrupting others and sitting still in the classroom. Most people in the United States value these traits, just as most disvalue the pain associated with physical illness. But because the values and expectations are not universally shared, controversies arise over these as well. For example, when critics question whether it is reasonable to expect all children to attend to classroom tasks, or whether there may be some benefit to the leaps of attention and thought characteristic of ADHD-diagnosable children, they are objecting to the values that make inattention and shifts in focus markers of dysfunction. One critical response, then, is to reject specific values associated with ADHD diagnostic criteria.

A broader argument suggests that ADHD is inappropriately understood as a disorder *of the individual*. Consider again the child whose behavior disrupts the classroom for his/her classmates. Often, such a child is not unhappy with his/her own behaviors and feelings—why, then, is that child medicated? Could there instead be a change in classroom structure, or others' expectations, to accommodate the behavior? More generally, the alternative proposed is that the social expectations of diagnosable children and adults is inflexible, or wrong, such that the "disorder" is more aptly described as a disorder of society than of the individual.

Conrad and Schneider also argue that the control of deviance with medical treatment is sometimes coercive.[18] As we have seen, although the values that determine what is considered mentally disordered (i.e., deviant) according to the standards of medical practice—and what must therefore be controlled—are widely shared, they are not entirely so, either within the medical profession or outside of it. Treatment, then, "...reinforces dominant values and adjusts people to their life situations (Conrad & Schneider, 1992 [1980], 242)."[19] On this view, for those who disagree with the dominant values, or whose life situation is undesirable on other grounds, altering the situation with treatment—rather than relaxing the values or altering the life situation—is coercive. The risk of coercion is increased by the high status of the medical professions relative to typical patients, and by the expert knowledge needed to be taken seriously in discourse concerning the definitions. According to anti-psychiatry psychiatrists Thomas Szasz and Sami Timimi, ADHD treatment is a case in point (Fulford, 2004; Schaler, 2004; Timimi, 2002). Avoiding coercion is, obviously, the option opened.

Related issues arises with respect to differences in behavioral expectations for boys/men and girls/women—a tangled set of considerations that has some arguing that ADHD differs across genders, others that it does not, and some arguing that ADHD is underdiagnosed in women, others that it is overdiagnosed across the board. But more background is required to adequately address these criticisms and the more general criticisms about medicalization and coercion. Later chapters discuss the sources of the contrasting values, and their consequences for the predominant view of ADHD and on ADHD-diagnosable people. Here, the availability of options to the current medical model is the primary point.

Biological vs. Social

As we have seen, the predominant concept of ADHD is that it is a biological phenomenon, the cause(s) of which will eventually be determined by scientific investigations. Clearly, biology *must* play a role in ADHD symptomatology, given that people are biological creatures: Biological-level interventions make sense in this context. Treatment patterns are also predictably focused on individual biology simply because intervening therapeutically with individuals' biology is the bulk of what physicians do and are trained to do. This is where their efficacy lies—they don't have control of school systems or workplace regulations, but they can offer assistance to the patient in their office. Aiding the individual, then—or, often in the case of ADHD, the family unit with which the physician also has contact—is a prime motivation for physicians' treatment decisions.

But Haslam's critique that ADHD lacks a latent structure joins others that question whether the current diagnostic structure of ADHD relevantly differentiates ADHD from "normal" or from other mental disorders. Chapter 2, which concerns the scientific study of ADHD, enumerates and discusses these issues, explaining how scientists have arrived at current conclusions and what gaps remain in present understanding. If the critics of the scientific status quo are right, then multiple alternative concepts open up, among them biological bases of dimensional models, primarily social models, psychodynamic models, developmental models emphasizing either social or physical influences, and various combinations of these.

The Drug Question

This topic, like the scientific controversies, requires more background and is taken up again in later chapters. Briefly, though, the current emphasis on medication as the primary treatment for ADHD (*see* Chapter 5 for details concerning the degree of emphasis) is tied closely to the predominant biological view. The exigencies of clinical practice also encourage this reliance—prescription medication is said to be more cost-effective than behavior management (Jensen et al., 2005)—an important pragmatic consideration. Critiques of pharmacotherapy come from a range of perspectives. Some object to the use of drugs, or to psychoactive drugs per se. Others tie their objections to arguments about coercion. Still others wonder about the drugs' efficacy (and therefore whether drug treatment is *really* cost effective). For example, abundant evidence indicates the short-term effectiveness of stimulants for behavior management, but only scant evidence exists for long-term effectiveness with goals such as academic or work achievement, despite the fact that many clinicians, caregivers, and ADHD-diagnosable individuals share a trust that medication helps achieve long-range goals. Safety concerns also continue, particularly ongoing evaluation of increased risk of cardiovascular events (U. S. Food and Drug Administration, 2010). As with other controversies, these criticisms suggest alternatives. Research might refocus, for example, to study a broader range of long-term results ("success" defined by various standards) and to develop strategies (pharmaceutical and otherwise, medical and otherwise) to achieve those successes safely.

Conclusion

The current view of ADHD—its internal complexity, and its relation to medical models of disease generally, to models of mental disorder, and the DSM's particular take on mental disorders—comprises a wealth of important decisions. Many of these are useful and endorsed, having been embraced by millions of diagnosable individuals and their physicians. However, many are controversial on empirical and value-based grounds. Empirical critique is discussed more fully in Chapter 2. Here, we have seen that the focus on biology, dysfunction, the individual, and categorical concepts has left the current model open to criticism that it problematically downplays context, complexity, and social bases for behaviors and interactions—in general, that it does not leave room for the multiple options still open for understanding and addressing problems currently associated with ADHD.

Describing these alternatives is not simply an academic exercise. Later chapters argue that the choices made in concepts and practice affect individuals and society more broadly—sometimes in negative ways. But before getting to those broader effects, we need more background. Medicine is not the only contributor to our present concepts of ADHD. Chapter 2 explores the contributions of the sciences to our current understanding.

REFERENCES

American Academy of Pediatrics: Committee on Quality Improvement, Subcommittee on Attention-Deficit/Hyperactivity Disorder (2001). Clinical practice guideline: treatment of the school-aged child with attention-deficit/hyperactivity disorder. *Pediatrics, 108*(4), 1033–1044.

American Academy of Child and Adolescent Psychiatry (2002). AACAP Official Action: Practice parameter for the use of stimulant medications in the treatment of children, adolescents, and adults. *Journal of the American Academy of Child and Adolescent Psychiatry, 41*(Suppl 2), 26S–49S.

American Psychiatric Association, Committee on Nomenclature and Statistics (1968). *Diagnostic and Statistical Manual of Mental Disorders, 2nd ed.* Washington, D.C.: American Psychiatric Association.

American Psychiatric Association (1980). *Diagnostic and Statistical Manual of Mental Disorders*, 3rd ed. Washington, D.C.: American Psychiatric Association.

American Psychiatric Association (1987). *Diagnostic and Statistical Manual of Mental Disorders*, 3rd ed., Rev. Washington, D.C.: American Psychiatric Association.

American Psychiatric Association (1994). *Diagnostic and Statistical Manual of Mental Disorders: DSM-IV*, 4 ed. Washington, DC: American Psychiatric Association.

American Psychiatric Association (2000). *Diagnostic and Statistical Manual of Mental Disorders* (4, Text Revision ed.). Arlington, VA: American Psychiatric Association.

American Psychiatric Association (2013). *Diagnostic and Statistical Manual of Mental Disorders: DSM-5* (5th ed.). Washington, DC: American Psychiatric Association.

Anonymous (2006). New data show adults continue to outpace children in growth of ADHD medication use. *Medco Media Room*, (March 21). Retrieved from http://medco.mediaroom.com/index.php?s=43&item=111

Baird, J., Stevenson, J. C., & Williams, D. C. (2000). The evolution of ADHD: a disorder of communication? *The Quarterly Review of Biology, 75*(1), 17–35.

Beauchamp, T. L., & Childress, J. F. (2001). *Priniciples of Biomedical Ethics* (5 ed.). New York: Oxford University Press.

Biederman, J., & Faraone, S. V. (2005). Attention-deficit hyperactivity disorder. *The Lancet, 366,* 237–248.

Biederman, J., Monuteaux, M. C., Mick, E., Spencer, T., Wilens, T. E., Silva, J. M., et al. (2006). Young adult outcome of attention deficit hyperactivity disorder: a controlled 10-year follow-up study. *Psychological Medicine, 36,* 167–179.

Boorse, C. (1975). On the distinction between disease and illness. *Philosophy and Public Affairs, 5,* 49–68.

Boorse, C. (1976). What a theory of mental health should be. *Journal for the Theory of Social Behaviour, 6*(1), 61–84.

Bouchard, M. F., Bellinger, D. C., Wright, R. O., & Weisskopf, M. G. (2010). Attention-deficit/hyperactivity disorder and urinary metabolites of organophosphate pesticides. *Pediatrics, 125*(6), e1270–e1277.

Brown, T. A., & Barlow, D. H. (2005). Dimensional versus categorical classification of mental disorders in the fifth edition of *Diagnostic and Statistical Manual of Mental Disorders* and beyond: comment on the special section. *Journal of Abnormal Psychology, 114*(4), 551–556.

Castellanos, F. X., & Tannock, R. (2002). Neuroscience of attention-deficit/hyperactivity disorder: the search for endophenotypes. *Nature Reviews: Neuroscience, 3*, 617–628.

Centers for Disease Control and Prevention (2005). Prevalence of diagnosis and medication treatment for attention-deficit/hyperactivity disorder—United States, 2003. *MMWR, 54*(34), 842–847.

Centers for Disease Control and Prevention (2012). 2011–2012 National Survey of Children's Health. Retrieved April 12, 2013, from http://www.cdc.gov/nchs/slaits/nsch.htm

Chai, G., Governale, L., McMahon, A. W., Trinidad, J. P., Staffa, J., & Murphy, D. (2012). Trends of outpatient prescription drug utilization in US children, 2002–2010. *Pediatrics, 130*(1), 23–31.

Clark, L. A. (2005). Temperament as a unifying basis for personality and psychopathology. *Journal of Abnormal Psychology, 114*(4), 505–521.

Colombo, A., Bendelow, G., Fulford, B., & Williams, S. (2003). Evaluating the influence of implicit models of mental disorder on processes of shared decision making within community-based multi-disciplinary teams. *Social Science and Medicine, 56*, 1557–1570.

Conrad, P., & Potter, D. (2000). From hyperactive child to ADHD adults: observations on the expansion of medical categories. *Social Problems, 47*(4), 559–582.

Conrad, P., & Schneider, J. W. (1992 [1980]). *Deviance and Medicalization: From Badness to Sickness*. Philadelphia, PA: Temple University Press.

Diller, L. H. (2006). *The Last Normal Child: Essays on the Intersection of Kids, Culture, and Psychiatric Drugs*. Westport, CT: Praeger Publishers.

Dopfner, M., Breuer, D., Wille, N., Erhart, M., & Ravens-Sieberer, U. (2008). How often do children meet ICD-10/DSM-IV criteria of attention deficit-/hyperactivity disorder and hyperkinetic disorder? Parent-based prevalence rates in a national sample—results of the BELLA study. *Eur Child Adolesc Psychiatry, 17*(Suppl 1), 59–70.

Eisenberg, L. (1972). Symposium: behavior modification by drugs. III. The clinical use of stimulant drugs in children. *Pediatrics, 49*(5), 709–715.

Elder, T. E. (2010). The importance of relative standards in ADHD diagnoses: evidence based on exact birth dates. *J Health Econ, 29*(5), 641–656.

Evans, W. N., Morrill, M. S., & Parente, S. T. (2010). Measuring inappropriate medical diagnosis and treatment in survey data: The case of ADHD among school-age children. *J Health Econ, 29*(5), 657–673.

First, M. B. (2005). Clinical utility: A prerequisite of the adoption of a dimensional approach in DSM. *Journal of Abnormal Psychology, 114*(4), 560–564.

Franke, B., Neale, B. M., & Faraone, S. V. (2009). Genome-wide association studies in ADHD. *Hum Genet, 126*(1), 13–50.

Froehlich, T. E., Lanphear, B. P., Auinger, P., Hornung, R., Epstein, J. N., Braun, J., et al. (2009). Association of tobacco and lead exposures with attention-deficit/hyperactivity disorder. *Pediatrics, 124*(6), e1054–e1063.

Froehlich, T. E., Lanphear, B. P., Epstein, J. N., Barbaresi, W. J., Katusic, S. K., & Kahn, R. S. (2007). Prevalence, recognition, and treatment of attention-deficit/hyperactivity disorder in a national sample of US children. *Archives of Pediatric and Adolescent Medicine, 161*(9), 857–864.

Fulford, K. W. M. (2004). Values-Based Medicine: Thomas Szasz's Legacy to Twenty-First Century Psychiatry. In J. A. Schaler (Ed.), *Szasz Under Fire: The Psychiatric Abolitionist Faces His Critics* (pp. 57–92). Chicago: Open Court.

Fulford, K. W. M., & Colombo, A. (2004). Six models of mental disorder: a study combining linguistic-analytic and empirical methods. *Philosophy, Psychiatry, and Psychology, 11*(2), 129–144.

Grady, D. L., Chi, H.-C., Ding, Y.-C., Smith, M., Wang, E., Schuck, S., et al. (2003). High prevalence of rare dopamine receptor D4 alleles in children diagnosed with attention-deficit hyperactivity disorder. *Molecular Psychiatry, 8*, 536–545.

Grinspoon, L., & Singer, S. B. (1973). Amphetamines in the treatment of hyperkinetic children. *Harvard Educational Review, 43*(4), 515–555.

Haslam, N. (2003). Kinds of kinds: a conceptual taxonomy of psychiatric categories. *Philosophy, Psychiatry, and Psychology, 9*(3), 203–217.

Haslam, N., Williams, B., Prior, M., Haslam, R., Graetz, B., & Sawyer, M. (2006). The latent structure of attention-deficit/hyperactivity disorder: a taxometric analysis. *Australian and New Zealand Journal of Psychiatry, 40*, 639–647.

Horwitz, A. V. (2002). *Creating Mental Illness*. Chicago: The University of Chicago Press.

Institute of Medicine, Division of Health Promotion and Disease Prevention (1992). The Second Fifty Years: Promoting Health and Preventing Disability. In R. L. Berg & J. S. Cassells (Eds.) Available August 18, 2006, from http://darwin.nap.edu/books/0309046815/html/22.html

Jensen, P. S., Garcia, J. A., Glied, S., Crowe, M., Foster, M., Schlander, M., et al. (2005). Cost-effectiveness of ADHD treatments: Findings from the Multimodal Treatment Study of Children with ADHD. *American Journal of Psychiatry, 162*(9), 1628–1636.

Kessler, R. C., Berglund, P., Demler, O., Jin, R., Merikangas, K. R., & Walters, E. E. (2005). Lifetime prevalence and age-of-onset distributions of DSM-IV disorders in the National Comorbidity Survey replication. *Archives of General Psychiatry, 62*, 593–602.

Krauch, V. (1971). Hyperactive engineering. *American Education, 7*, 12–16.

Kupfer, D. J. (2005). Dimensional models for research and diagnosis: a current dilemma. *Journal of Abnormal Psychology, 114*(4), 557–559.

Lahey, B. B., Applegate, B., McBurnett, K., Biederman, J., Greenhill, L., Hynd, G. W., et al. (1994). DSM-IV field trials for attention deficit hyperactivity disorder in children and adolescents. *American Journal of Psychiatry, 151*(11), 1673–1685.

Langley, K., Marshall, L., van den Bree, M., Thomas, H., Owen, M., O'Donovan, M., et al. (2004). Association of the dopamine D4 receptor gene 7-repeat allele with neuropsychological test performance of children with ADHD. *American Journal of Psychiatry, 161*(1), 133–138.

Linnet, K. M., Wisborg, K., Obel, C., Secher, N. J., Thomsen, P. H., Agerbo, E., et al. (2005). Smoking during pregnancy and the risk for hyperkinetic disorder in offspring. *Pediatrics, 116*(2), 462–466.

Lunbeck, E. (1994). *The Psychiatric Persuasion: Knowledge, Gender, and Power in Modern America*. Princeton, NJ: Princeton University Press.

Mayes, R., Bagwell, C., & Erkulwater, J. (2009). *Medicating Children: ADHD and Pediatric Mental Health*. Cambridge, MA: Harvard University Press.

Mayes, S. D., Calhoun, S. L., & Crowell, E. W. (2000). Learning disabilities and ADHD: Overlapping spectrum disorders. *Journal of Learning Disabilities, 33*(5), 417–424.

McCracken, J. T. (2000). Chapter 39.1. Attention-deficit disorders. In B. J. Sadock & V. A. Sadock (Eds.), *Kaplan & Sadock's Comprehensive Textbook of Psychiatry* (7 ed., Vol. 2, pp. 2679–2688). Philadelphia, PA: Lippincott Williams & Wilkins.

Megone, C. (2000). Mental illness, human function, and values. *Philosophy, Psychiatry, and Psychology, 7*(1), 45–65.

Merikangas, K. R., He, J. P., Brody, D., Fisher, P. W., Bourdon, K., & Koretz, D. S. (2010). Prevalence and treatment of mental disorders among US children in the 2001–2004 NHANES. *Pediatrics, 125*(1), 75–81.

Miller, F. (1973). Getting Billy into the game. *American Education, 9*, 22–27.

Murphy, D., & Woolfolk, R. L. (2001). The harmful dysfunction analysis of mental disorder. *Philosophy, Psychiatry, and Psychology, 7*(4), 241–252.

National Center for Health Statistics (2006). *Health, United States, 2006, with Chartbook on Trends in the Health of Americans*. Hyattsville, MD: U.S. Government Printing Office.

National Institutes of Health (1998). *Diagnosis and treatment of attention deficit hyperactivity disorder (ADHD): NIH Consensus Statement*. Bethesda, Maryland: National Institutes of Health.

Neuman, R. J., Todd, R. D., Heath, A. C., Reich, W., Hudziak, J. J., Bucholz, K. K., et al. (1999). Evaluation of ADHD typology in three contrasting samples: a latent class approach. *Journal of the American Academy of Child and Adolescent Psychiatry, 38*(1), 25–33.

Nigg, J. T., Blaskey, L. G., Huang-Pollock, C. L., Hinshaw, S. P., John, O. P., Willcutt, E. G., et al. (2002). Big five dimensions and ADHD symptoms: links between personality traits and clinical symptoms. *Journal of Personality and Social Psychology*, 83(2), 451–469.

Nigg, J. T., Nikolas, M., Mark Knottnerus, G., Cavanagh, K., & Friderici, K. (2010). Confirmation and extension of association of blood lead with attention-deficit/hyperactivity disorder (ADHD) and ADHD symptom domains at population-typical exposure levels. *J Child Psychol Psychiatry*, 51(1), 58–65.

Ogdie, M. N., Macphie, L., Minassian, S. L., Yang, M., Fisher, S. E., Francks, C., et al. (2003). A genomewide scan for attention-deficit/hyperactivity disorder in an extended sample: suggestive linkage on 17p11. *American Journal of Human Genetics*, 72, 1268–1279.

PDM Task Force (2006). *Psychodynamic Diagnostic Manual*. Silver Springs, MD: Alliance of Psychoanalytic Organizations.

Peterson, S., Shulman, S., & Ireys, H. (2007). *Quality care for children with ADHD: the role of primary care physicians*. Washington, D.C.: Mathematica Policy Research, Inc. (under contract with the Health Resources and Services Administration, U.S. Department of Health and Human Services).

Pliszka, S., Bernet, W., Bukstein, O., Walter, H. J., Arnold, V., Beitchman, J., et al. (2007). Practice parameter for the assessment and treatment of children and adolescents with attention-deficit/hyperactivity disorder *Journal of the American Academy of Child and Adolescent Psychiatry*, 46(7), 894–921.

Rafalovich, A. (2004). *Framing ADHD Children: A Critical Examination of the History, Discourse, and Everyday Experience of Attention Deficit/Hyperactivity Disorder*. Lanham, MD: Lexington Books.

Reznek, L. (1991). *The Philosophical Defence of Psychiatry*. London: Routledge.

Sax, L., & Kautz, K. J. (2003). Who first suggests the diagnosis of attention-deficit/hyperactivity disorder? *Annals of Family Medicine*, 1(3), 171–174.

Schaler, J. A. (Ed.). (2004). *Szasz Under Fire: The Psychiatric Abolitionist Faces His Critics* (Vol. 1). Chicago: Open Court.

Schwartz, P. H. (2007). Defining dysfunction: natural selection, design, and drawing a line. *Philosophy of Science*, 74, 364–385.

Shaw, P., Eckstrand, K., Sharp, W., Blumenthal, J., Lerch, J. P., Greenstein, D., et al. (2007). Attention-deficit/hyperactivity disorder is characterized by a delay in cortical maturation. *Proceedings of the National Academy of Science*, 104(49), 19,649–19,654.

Swing, E. L., Gentile, D. A., Anderson, C. A., & Walsh, D. A. (2010). Television and video game exposure and the development of attention problems. *Pediatrics*, 126(2), 214–221.

Timimi, S. (2002). *Pathological Child Psychiatry and the Medicalization of Childhood*. East Sussex, UK: Brunner-Routledge.

Tripp, G., & Wickens, J. R. (2009). Neurobiology of ADHD. *Neuropharmacology*, 57(7–8), 579–589.

U.S. Food and Drug Administration. (2010). Communication about an Ongoing Safety Review of Stimulant Medications used in Children with Attention-Deficit/

Hyperactivity Disorder (ADHD). Retrieved January 15, 2010, from http://www.fda.gov/Drugs/DrugSafety/PostmarketDrugSafetyInformationforPatientsandProviders/DrugSafetyInformationforHeathcareProfessionals/ucm165858.htm

Wakefield, J. C. (2002). Values and the Validity of Diagnostic Criteria: Disvalued versus Disordered Conditions of Childhood and Adolescence. In J. Z. Sadler (Ed.), *Descriptions and Prescriptions: Values, Mental Disorders, and the DSMs* (pp. 148–164). Baltimore, MD: The Johns Hopkins University Press.

Widiger, T. A., & Samuel, D. B. (2005). Diagnostic categories or dimensions? A question for the *Diagnostic and Statistical Manual of Mental Disorders—Fifth Edition. Journal of Abnormal Psychology, 114*(4), 494–504.

World Health Organization (2002). *Towards a Common Language for Functioning, Disability, and Health: ICF: The International Classification of Functioning, Disability, and Health*. Geneva: World Health Organization.

Zarin, D. A., Tanielian, T. L., Suarez, A. P., & Marcus, S. C. (1998). Datapoints: treatment of attention-deficit hyperactivity disorder by different physician specialties. *Psychiatric Services, 49*, 171. Retrieved October 17, 2007, from http://psychservices.psychiatryonline.org/cgi/content/full/49/2/171

Zito, J. M., Safer, D. J., dosReis, S., Magder, L. S., Gardner, J. F., & Zarin, D. A. (1999). Psychotherapeutic medication patterns for youths with attention-deficit/hyperactivity disorder. *Archives of Pediatric and Adolescent Medicine, 153*(12), 1257–1263.

Zoler, M. L. (2010). Prevalence of ADHD in U.S. youths reached 9.5% in 2007–2008. *Internal Medicine News Digital Network*. Retrieved January 27, 2011, from http://www.internalmedicinenews.com/index.php?id=495&cHash=071010&tx_ttnews[tt_news]=18359

NOTES

1. Throughout, I use the term "values" broadly, to include pragmatic interests as well as ethical values.
2. The 2013 DSM-5 criteria are discussed in Chapter 6.
3. Interpolating from data provided by for 1995 and 2002 time points, there were approximately 175,000,000 office visits for those under 18 in 1998. (National Center for Health Statistics, 2006)
4. The remainder represented a variety of other referral sources.
5. Global Sales of ADHD drugs were forecasted to reach US $4.3 billion by 2012–Market research available on CNS drug discoveries 2006: Attention Deficit Hyperactivity Disorder Posted on: Friday, December 15, 2006, 09:01 CST, http://www.redorbit.com/news/health/768760/global_sales_of_adhd_drugs_are_forecast_to_reach_us43/index.html. Accessed February 13, 2010.
6. The DSM-5 definition of mental disorder differs in some ways from the DSM-IV definition, but the key points of the analysis in this and later chapters still hold.

7. The categorical criterion is not as unsubtle as it sounds in this description; I provide more detail in Part 2.
8. The study was done in the United Kingdom; its purpose was to identify models of mental disorder used by the various groups, and to interpret how these might affect power relations and communication in multidisciplinary teams, with a longer-range goal of enhancing the abilities of multidisciplinary teams to provide patient care. Given that diagnosis and medication rates for ADHD are lower in the United Kingdom than in the United States (i.e., that there is less evidence of adherence to a medical model in that aspect of practice in the United Kingdom than in the United States), I do not think Fulford and Colombo's conclusions overstate the case for psychiatry's assumptions in the United States.
9. In 1976, the journal *School Review* devoted an issue to this topic (Vol. 85:1).
10. "Operations" and "mechanisms" also produce something of interest and therefore do not shed the value-valence. The definition is circular, but that reinforces the point.
11. Another important argument against Wakefield's view is that many cognitive functions relevant to mental health may not be designed by evolution but may instead be "spandrels"—side effects of other traits that were shaped by evolution. They would therefore be valued for anthropocentric, not evolutionary, reasons. (Murphy & Woolfolk, 2001)
12. It is somewhat ambiguous what Schwartz means by "value judgments." I take him to mean not subjective judgments, but judgments made in accord with a set of values.
13. In the articles cited, First and Kupfer argue in *favor* of categorical dimensions for the upcoming DSM-5, but they nicely summarize arguments on the opposing side.
14. It is worth noting that conceiving of disorders categorically is consistent with holding that there are variations of severity within the category, and with observations that some individuals nearly or partially meet the criteria; these "shades of gray" are often important clinically. Such judgments are built into the diagnostic criteria, in that symptoms must have been present "to a degree that is maladaptive," and treatment protocols also take severity and comorbidities into account. Critics of categorical classification find this clinical finessing inadequate, however.
15. Haslam et al. also argue, but did not test taxometrically, that the existence of subtypes is unlikely in the absence of a type (Haslam, William et al., 2006).
16. The empirical debates are discussed in more detail in Chapter 2.
17. The disagreement between psychodynamic vs. organic approaches to diagnosis has several generations of tradition behind it. Historian Elizabeth Lunbeck discusses the difference in terms of early twentieth century dynamic psychiatrists' reaction to the organic focus of Kraepelin, called by some the "father of modern psychiatry." Not so, according to the dynamic psychiatrists. "Dynamic

psychiatrists would spurn diagnosis in favor of attention to the 'whole person' and his or her fit to the environment. Focus on disease entities—schizophrenia, for example—split the patient into too many parts, they argued, and made the disease, not the patient, the object of attention" (Lunbeck, 1994, 118).
18. Recalling that drawing a line marking dysfunction requires a normative element, we can see why critics more pointedly use the term "deviance" to describe the differences picked out by (at least some) DSM norms.
19. Conrad and Schneider specify psychotherapy in the full quote, but I hazard that today they would include pharmacological treatment as well.

2 HOW SCIENCE SHAPES ADHD

Scientists propose multiple hypotheses to explain ADHD-associated traits and behaviors, their causes and mechanisms, their treatment and prognosis. Some of the hypotheses conflict with DSM-defined criteria (American Psychiatric Association, 2000; American Psychiatric Association, 2013), but the sciences (to date) have remained committed to models that align with DSM-defined ADHD. Why? In part, of course, because the data fit the DSM criteria to some extent. Useful literature reviews suggest that this is the case (Castellanos, Kelly, & Milham, 2009; Dopheide & Pliszka, 2009; Mayes, Bagwell, & Erkulwater, 2009; Singh, 2008; Taylor, 2009; Tripp & Wickens, 2009), weighing evidence in favor of and against various underlying mechanisms for DSM-defined ADHD.

A different perspective, though, reveals additional reasons that the sciences of ADHD continue, for the most part, to accept the predominant model. Simultaneously, the shift in views clarifies factors that can support less-examined alternatives. To establish the alternative viewpoints, this chapter examines science's commitments to certain reasoning patterns and methodologies. The first section introduces common reasoning patterns in the sciences, such as achieving interlevel explanations, demonstrating data convergence, understanding mechanisms, and reducing explanations to ever-finer biological levels. Given gaps in current empirical data, these reasoning patterns allow much room for interpretation and alternatives, rather than driving to particular conclusions. The second section argues that despite the room for alternatives, the typical reasoning patterns, together with more specific statistical and practical methodological choices, have helped shape the understanding of ADHD to its current form. Recent results in genetics, diverse hypotheses in neurophysiology, and heterogeneity in clinical presentation and response all threaten to fragment the predominant model. Yet the epistemic and methodological factors contribute to keeping the present view of ADHD in place despite conflicting data and available alternatives.

Reasoning Patterns in ADHD Sciences

Varied Fields, Unifying Goals

Many fields study ADHD, but surveying the ADHD literature makes the biological focus in the research clear. In a random sample of 150 articles on ADHD drawn from a wide range of journals, 58% expressed a primarily biological view of ADHD's etiology, 10% specified a mixed understanding (for example, gene–environment interaction), and in 19% the etiological understanding was ambiguous. Only a few articles (7%) suggested that the authors held an alternative view or at least had an alternative emphasis in their research: seven measured primarily behavioral parameters; two measured psychosocial parameters; two focused on communication; and none on education. (Nine articles were omitted from the analysis because they were not available online.)[1]

The predominant biological orientation of ADHD research represents work in fields such as biological psychiatry, psychopharmacology, behavioral and molecular genetics, and the clinical sciences affiliated with psychiatry, psychology, neurology, pediatrics, and epidemiology. Other, not necessarily biologically oriented, contributing sciences include cognition-oriented branches of psychology, along with social sciences such as anthropology, social psychology, and educational psychology.

These sciences are diverse, and their goals, research methods, and data assessment criteria vary. Still, one can observe common ground in their approaches. At a very general level, each is committed to some version of "the" scientific method—that is, to being able to demonstrate results by means of experiment or observation. In turn, this very general commitment reflects a view that phenomena can be explained by reference only to physical entities, as opposed to metaphysical, spiritual, magical, vitalistic, psychological, or otherwise nonphysical entities. The sciences also commit to their own fallibility—current ideas considered good-enough-for-now, in full knowledge that hypotheses can be disproven, theories overturned, and better ideas will come along.

Types of Studies

Across the sciences, studies of ADHD fall into three general categories: descriptive, mechanism-seeking, and therapeutic. Descriptive research aims to refine the understanding of ADHD's phenomenology without expressly seeking mechanisms or causes for the trait, behavior, or other correlate the scientist is interested in. For example, psychologists might observe childhood behaviors, social circumstances, ADHD types, or comorbidities to see if any of these predict a later outcome such as level of academic achievement (Barry, Lyman, & Klinger, 2002; Braaten et al., 2003; Mayes, Calhoun, & Crowell, 2000; Ohan & Johnston, 2007; Ostrander, Crystal, & August, 2006); epidemiologists might correlate an environmental exposure, such as lead exposure or television viewing, with ADHD prevalence (Christakis, Zimmerman, DiGiuseppe, & McCarty, 2004; Swing, Gentile, Anderson, & Walsh, 2010; Woodruff et al., 2004); or teams might seek differences between ADHD-diagnosable and non-diagnosable individuals' brains (Dimoska, Johnstone, Barry, & Clarke, 2003; Durston et al., 2004). The second research category seeks mechanisms that underlie and explain the observed phenomena. The majority of research in this category seeks neuroanatomic or molecular mechanisms, including actions of "susceptibility genes," neurotransmitters, excitation patterns, or neural pathways (Franke, Neale, & Faraone, 2009; Gizer, Ficks, & Waldman, 2009; Terje Sagvolden, Aase, Johansen, & Russell, 2005; Tripp & Wickens, 2009). The therapeutic strand of research explores interventions such as pharmaceutical treatment, behavior therapy, classroom modification, training of slow cortical potentials, and many other possibilities (Anhalt, McNeil, & Bahl, 1998; Heinrich, Gevensleben, Freislander, Moll, & Rothenberger, 2004; Miranda & Presentacion, 2000; Pelham & Fabiano, 2008; Spencer et al., 2001).

These research categories, pursued by diverse sciences, are mutually supportive in part because they all take their object of inquiry to be the same thing: DSM-defined ADHD. They also raise new questions for one another: Descriptions or therapeutic success can fuel a search for mechanisms, and understanding mechanisms can lead to new phenomena to describe or new possibilities for intervention. These aspects of mutual support are just two elements of the conceptual "glue" holding diverse findings together.

Generalizations

One of the most common reasoning patterns in biology, medicine, and psychology is the framing of generalizations. An old-fashioned view holds that scientists aim to discover laws of nature—generalizations that apply universally and invariantly. However, philosophers of biology, philosophers of social science, and scientists themselves have long recognized that this view of science does not describe the practices or goals of sciences involving living things (*see*, e.g., Beatty, 1995; Schaffner, 1993). Living systems (such as organisms, species, or ecosystems) are generally too complex and subject to too many variables for strictly invariant laws to be demonstrated. In addition, a phenomenon may be isolated to a small number of individuals, species, or systems, so that finding generalizations that apply universally may not be a relevant goal. Instead, the goal in the life sciences is empirically demonstrated generalizations with an appropriate *scope,* and within that scope, greater or lesser *invariance* (Woodward, 2000).[2]

The standards for scope and invariance vary, depending on the subject of the generalization, the purpose to which it is put, and the science's level of development. For example, a drug for widespread use must be near-universally nontoxic (within prescribing limits)—that is, the generalization "drug X is nontoxic" must be highly invariant and have broad scope. However, some variation in efficacy is typically tolerable: For example, the generalization "atomoxetine is effective" is considered true when the drug benefits 45% of patients (Spencer, 2009)—that is, a moderately invariant generalization is acceptable.

Room for Debate

The categorical model of ADHD, in which people either have ADHD or do not, embeds the generalization "people who meet ADHD diagnostic criteria differ qualitatively from those who do not." But, in the literature of the ADHD sciences, a frequent critique is that this and many finer generalizations are *too* broad, glossing over extensive variability among diagnosable and nondiagnosable people (Bush, 2010; Gizer et al., 2009; Parens & Johnston, 2009; Sonuga-Barke & Castellanos, 2005). (We will see in Part 2 that recent research is beginning to address this critique directly.) Criticisms of the current predominant model that are based on this point do not object to the scientific practice of generalizing per se, but instead demand higher standards for defensible generalizations. Such critique leaves open the possibility that different generalizations might better fit the existing data.

Interlevel Reasoning

Scientists, like the rest of us, can examine and explain events or phenomena in different ways. An ornithologist might say that a bird cracked open a seed because its muscles contracted and relaxed in a specific sequence, because its brain signaled its muscles to initiate the sequence, or because it had been trained to do so—each of these suggestions explains the event differently, but the explanations are not contradictory. Instead, each focuses on a different level[3] of explanation—describable as physiological, neurological, and behavioral—and the answers may well be complementary. However, the explanations, examined more carefully, answer different questions: What made the motion possible? What initiated the motion? Why did the bird move at the time it did? Detailed research on each of these questions would involve different expertise on the scientist's part, and no single scientist or research program would be likely to investigate all three. Still, the ornithologists would all see their results as contributing to the understanding of feeding behavior.

Similarly, the sciences that study ADHD vary greatly in the questions they ask and in the level to which they direct those questions. ADHD-relevant traits, behaviors, events, or correlates can be described at psychological or cognitive, behavioral, relational, or social levels. Biologically oriented research can target varied levels: molecular, subcellular, cellular, cell network, whole organ, whole organism, and organism/environment interaction. Any of these levels might be relevant to ADHD's etiology, expression, or management, and scientists work at each level. As with the bird case, an explanation for an ADHD-associated behavior—say, not staying seated in class—might take many forms: a genetic propensity, hypoactive dopamine circuits, overstimulation (or boredom) in the classroom environment, and so forth. Once again, these varying responses answer different questions: What makes a child more likely to express this behavior? What maintains the tendency to express this behavior? Why do children express this behavior in class? As in the bird case, these varying questions and explanations need not conflict and may be complementary. Again similarly, each answer is interpreted as contributing to the science of ADHD.

Notice, too, that the explanandum—that is, the thing to be explained—is also at a particular level—in the example just given, at the behavioral level. That means that an explanation involving other levels—genes, dopamine, neural pathways, or the social setting—provides an *interlevel* explanation of the behavior: A phenomenon at one level is explained by mechanisms or circumstances at another level. Interlevel explanations, although not universal in science, are very typical in the sciences that study ADHD. Indeed, it is quite common for researchers to attempt to link several levels in their explanations, often in complex ways. For example, one paper links the low-level neurophysiology of dopamine through successive levels of behavioral intervention studies in rats and children, parenting styles, and "real-world" outcomes, culminating in high-level cultural expectations (in my reconstruction of their argument, which follows, a "finding" is a conclusion of a previous study, a "hypothesis" is the authors' prediction for future studies, based on the stated findings and others) (Sagvolden et al., 2005):

Finding 1: In rats, reinforcement of behavior is associated with increased activity in the brain's mesolimbic dopamine system.

Assumption 1: Rat neurophysiology and behavior are relevantly similar to human neurophysiology and behavior.

Finding(s) 2: Dopamine is involved in ADHD-drug function, ADHD genetics, and the neurophysiology of mood, memory, and behavior.

Hypothesis 2: Decreased activity in the mesolimbic dopamine system contributes to ADHD-associated undesired behaviors.

Hypothesis 3: With decreased activity in the mesolimbic dopamine system, immediate, repeated, and consistent feedback is needed to reinforce desired behaviors.

Finding 3: Clinical research suggests that immediate, repeated, and consistent feedback increases desired behavior in children who have ADHD.

Finding 4: For children who have ADHD, an impulsive, disorganized, and inconsistent upbringing is correlated with a grave outcome.

Hypothesis 4: Lack of immediate, repeated, and consistent feedback is one feature of an impulsive, disorganized, and inconsistent upbringing. This feature, and its underlying neurobiology, explains the correlation in Finding 4.

Hypothesis 5: Cultures with strict expectations for children's behavior, in which parents provide immediate, repeated, and consistent feedback from early childhood, may have fewer children who exhibit ADHD-associated behaviors.

The lower-level neurophysiological findings in rats and humans (Findings 1 and 2, among others not stated) lead Sagvolden et al. to propose a lower-level mechanism for ADHD (Hypothesis 2). Building on this, successive higher-level links of findings and hypotheses can then explain higher-level grave outcomes for some ADHD-diagnosable children (Hypothesis 4) and make a higher-level cross-cultural prediction (Hypothesis 5). The interlevel reasoning works in concert with other patterns discussed below: convergence of evidence (from various types of studies, and various fields), analogy (rats to humans), and mechanistic reasoning (an available mechanism reinforces the relevance of the findings to the hypotheses). Importantly, interlevel reasoning requires that categories and terms be defined similarly within and across fields; this requires consistent operationalization (*see* below).

Room for Debate

It can be difficult to determine the point at which evidence adequately supports an interlevel theory. Sagvolden et al.'s theory is certainly plausible, for example. But consider the point I've called "Hypothesis 4." A correlation between impulsive, disorganized, and inconsistent upbringing and grave outcomes for children who have ADHD has been observed. But there might be reasons for this other than lower dopamine activity and inadequate reinforcement schedules. ADHD-diagnosable children have multiple comorbidities—depression, other behavior disorders, learning disabilities—perhaps these are involved. Or multiple pathways and mechanisms, rather than simply the dopamine system, might be needed to explain the effect. That is, ample room remains, in this example, for alternative hypotheses.[4]

Operationalization

To report their data, scientists need to clarify just what it is they are observing. That is, they need to *operationalize* the phenomenon of interest by describing precisely what observations they will make or measurements they will take to represent it. A scientist who wants to study drug effects on "growth" in ADHD-diagnosed children might measure their heights, comparing heights of those who have and have not taken methylphenidate. Weight could provide an alternative or additional measure, as could some less-typical operationalization, such as circumference of a specific body region. Often, operationalizations are more complex, as when scientists study objects or events that are too small, too far away, or too poorly defined to have an obvious measurement. In the case of unobservables, researchers often presume (for good reasons) that effects stem from the activity of physical entities, but they do not observe the entities themselves. Electroencephalograms (EEGs) operationalize patterns of electrical activity in the brain, and "brain scans," such as functional MRI and PET, operationalize metabolic activity; neither the electrical activity nor the metabolic activity is observed directly. In many cases, the appropriate operationalization is not obvious, and choices may be readily disputed. For example, if Sagvolden et al. chose to investigate their "Hypothesis 4," above, they would need to state how they would define and measure "immediate, repeated, and consistent feedback," "impulsive, disorganized, and inconsistent upbringing," and "grave outcome." Clearly, different scientists would be able to choose different (reasonable) measurements representing these rather vague descriptors. The ADHD diagnostic criteria are themselves used as an operationalization that defines the choice of the study group.

Operationalization *filters* observations by making certain observations relevant to a conclusion and others irrelevant. For this reason, a change in operationalization has the potential to change outcomes. For example, to measure ADHD "treatment success," Jensen et al. used "...a combined overall rating, completed by both parents and teachers, of DSM-IV symptoms of ADHD and oppositional defiant disorder, using the SNAP scale, developed by Swanson and colleagues (Jensen et al., 2005, 1629)." What would happen if the research team instead operationalized "treatment success" in terms of life satisfaction? Satterfield et al. operationalized "criminality" as "evaluation of adolescent and official adult arrest records (Satterfield & Schell, 1997, 1728)." Would measuring "criminality" by counting prison terms significantly alter their conclusions?

Room for Debate

Deciding what operationalizations are appropriate arouses much debate. In addition, the practices of operationalizing and indirect observation introduce tensions between practice and basic commitments in science. First, the construct represented by the operationalization can be confused with the physical entities that produce it: "intelligence," "ADHD," or "lighting up on MRI" can incorrectly be equated with physical properties of the brain or brain function in an error of *reification*. Scientists understand that reification is unsupportable; nevertheless, the tendency—although not universal—persists. (*See* below for a discussion of reasons for the persistence.) Second, operationalization introduces nonphysical elements to scientific conclusions. For example, choosing specific measurements to stand in for admired traits such as "intelligence" or "efficacy" or to represent concerns about "grave outcomes" or "ADHD" draws in the values underlying the admiration or concern. The second point is important to the conclusions in Chapters 4 and 5.

Convergence

In interpreting their own results, researchers often draw on and connect evidence from multiple experiments that use a variety of techniques across many levels and in many disciplines. Convergence of the varied data helps make scientific reasoning convincing. Philosopher Susan Haack likens this aspect of scientific reasoning to filling in a crossword puzzle. As one skillfully fills in squares, the penciled-in letters limit the choices for the remaining squares, and the possibility that *all* the squares are wrong grows dimmer (Haack, 1995). Scientists "fill in" the links they need between ideas in various ways. Direct empirical demonstration is one strategy, as are different kinds of reasoning (inductive, deductive, abductive, statistical, etc.), that rely to various degrees on assumptions and empirical demonstration. Sometimes authors are explicit about this using convergence. Durston et al. argue that, "*Converging evidence* implies the involvement of dopaminergic frontostriatal circuitry in ADHD (Durston et al., 2003), 871, italics added)," going on to cite numerous articles with which their findings are "consistent" or "in line." In the example detailed above, Sagvolden et al. point out consistencies between pharmacological research in humans, studies of molecular and neural activity in rats, and behavioral and sociological studies in children (Sagvolden et al., 2005).

Room for Debate

Convergences claimed in scientific reasoning can be more or less watertight. In the example from Sagvolden et al., Hypothesis 2—although it relies on indirect evidence such as pharmaceutical effectiveness—requires fewer links across experiment types, fields, and levels than Hypothesis 5. Both hypotheses are contested, but Hypothesis 2 avoids, among other potential "missing links," any weaknesses in Hypotheses 3 and 4. Challenging other scientists' links is part of the process of science.

Analogy

Sagvolden et al.'s Hypothesis 1 employs an aspect of convergent reasoning that deserves special attention—the linking of animal research to findings in humans. For practical and ethical reasons, scientists conduct much work in biomedical science using animals ("animal models") rather than human subjects. As the example illustrates, a key claim in study of mental disorders is that an animal model of a human disorder "is like" a human disorder, because an experimental animal "is like" a person.[5] The animal model:human "link" is made by analogy.

Room for Debate

An animal model:human analogy can be better or worse.[6] Animal models for ADHD are highly contentious. Against Sagvolden's model, for example, Rubia argues that rats and people are poorly homologous for conditions involving cognition, given rats' "... nearly inexistent frontal lobes and reduced number of complex neural networks... (Rubia, 2005, 439)." Karatekin (2005) argues that reinforcement is a much more complex and variable phenomenon in humans than in rats (or pigeons). Sagvolden et al. (2009) counter that their ADHD model organism, the spontaneously hypertensive rat, is relevantly similar in behavior, responses to behavioral conditioning, and gene expression to children with hyperactive-impulsive type and combined-type ADHD. They propose that a different rat breed be used for modeling inattentive-type ADHD.

Mechanism

Even with gaps in interlevel explanations filled in with convergences and analogy, however, the forms of reasoning so far discussed leave out a central scientific goal: explanations based on mechanisms. A clear and complete mechanistic explanation requires that mechanisms at each level, as well as mechanisms of interaction among levels, be empirically demonstrated. The complexity of the systems involved in ADHD mediate against this; still, the more detailed the story, the clearer the mechanistic explanation.

As discussed previously, much ADHD research studies underlying biology. Biologically oriented research may be primarily descriptive, and very often, as in pharmacological research, its overarching goal is intervention. Many such studies, though, aim for better comprehension of the mechanisms underlying ADHD-associated traits and behaviors. Scientists often find that even studies that are primarily descriptive contribute to this goal—for example, when functional magnetic resonance imaging (fMRI) shows that the ventral striatum is differently active in ADHD-diagnosable and typical brains during an assigned task in which subjects expect a reward (Durston, 2008), the descriptive finding contributes to the hypothesis that the ventral striatum is involved in a mechanism associated with ADHD symptomatology.[7] Conversely, study of mechanisms often drives new possibilities for intervention and reveals new phenomena for description.

Philosophers of science debate the definition of "mechanism."[8] Most of this discussion is not crucial to this chapter. One issue that will concern us, however, is whether the goal of elucidating mechanisms is *reductionistic*; this topic is taken up in Part 2. For this reason, I focus here on William Bechtel's definition for "mechanism," which (later) grounds an argument that search for mechanisms is *not* reductionistic; I will disagree, and will argue in contrast that the ADHD sciences as a whole *are* reductionistic. According to Bechtel, "A mechanism is a structure performing a function in virtue of its component parts, component operations, and their organization. The orchestrated functioning of the mechanism is responsible for one or more phenomena (Bechtel, 2008, 13)." This view of mechanisms specifies that they are physical objects (component parts) that, when arranged in a certain pattern (their organization) and undergoing certain processes or changes (component operations), result in the objects performing a function that results in (observable) phenomena. Component parts' relevance depends on the phenomenon of interest, so that mechanisms can explain phenomena occurring at various levels, including psychological, behavioral, and social as well as biological and chemical levels. Mechanisms explaining higher-level phenomena are, of course, immensely complex: If scientists wished to detail a mechanism underlying ADHD-diagnosable children's relative unpopularity with peers, they would need, in stages and with multiple techniques, to demonstrate relevant processes at many levels, as well as the parts and operations linking the processes. In the interim, they would seek a tight set of correlations that might yield such detail after further study.[9] In the earlier example, Sagvolden et al. hypothesize such interlocking connections to explain the phenomenon that disorganized parenting correlates with poor outcome.

Room for Debate

Basic scientists in ADHD research concur that no one has yet adequately elucidated the mechanism(s) for ADHD-related phenomena. A review by several prominent ADHD researchers puts the point as follows: "Thus while the field has reached a point at which relatively sophisticated causal theories are proposed...we remain some distance from demonstrating a full causal model of ADHD, or its component symptom dimensions, in a way that incorporates multiple levels of analysis" (Coghill, Nigg, Rothenberger, Sonuga-Barke, & Tannock, 2005,105).

Some Key Debates

As we have just seen, important reasoning patterns in the sciences leave room for ambiguities and alternative interpretations within the sciences of ADHD. The nature of most disagreement among scientists is non-radical in that it remains consistent with scientists' commitments to the reasoning patterns described above. In addition, although researchers propose varying hypotheses about ADHD's etiology, most ADHD science remains committed to the predominant understanding of ADHD simply by virtue of taking the DSM model as an object of inquiry. Similarly, some degree of concern about the current category's heterogeneity and comorbidities is consistent with a need to refine rather than reject the category.

Nevertheless, some scientific critique threatens to dislodge current understanding of ADHD. Chapter 1 discussed criticisms of the DSM's categorical understanding of ADHD. More far-reaching than it might at first appear, this criticism affects not only concepts of disorder but also hypotheses about ADHD's etiology. As Haslam et al. (2006) put it:

> The categorical view, embodied in diagnostic systems such as the DSM-IV, holds that affected and unaffected individuals differ qualitatively, separated by a non-arbitrary category boundary. Accordingly, aetiological models should invoke causal factors that are specific to affected individuals and capable of generating a discontinuity. On the continuum view, ADHD falls at the end of a seamless trait distribution, differing from normality only by degree. (p. 639).

If the "continuum view" is correct, causes would likely be multifactorial and interactive, no distinctive neurophysiological trait would be identifiable, and ADHD would simply be a pragmatic diagnosis, rather than having a distinctive biological etiology like many diseases. Other authors suggest that the DSM is mistaken in lumping the subtypes of ADHD under one diagnostic category; instead, they argue, inattentive forms of ADHD differ from hyperactive/impulsive forms etiologically as well as in overt behavior (Sagvolden et al., 2005; Sagvolden et al., 2009). Some etiological hypotheses have similarly far-reaching potential to change current views and practices. Views that ADHD represents delayed but otherwise normal development (Shaw et al., 2007), if demonstrated to be correct, might change the propensity to term ADHD a disorder. Etiological hypotheses that stress environmental effects or gene–environment interactions, if demonstrated to be as significant or more significant than current neurotransmitter-centered hypotheses, might refocus responses from pharmacological intervention to preventive efforts.

In short, the DSM model of ADHD is not the only scientifically plausible model, as scientific methods—and debates within the scientific community—clearly show.

Structure by Choice

Despite the controversies, ambiguities, and alternatives, however, key aspects of the DSM-defined model of ADHD continue to hold. For over 30 years, the categorical conception and the behavioral traits of interest have been relatively constant. General aspects of the etiological hypotheses, such as the involvement of monoamines and high heritability suggesting genetic influences, have remained stable over a somewhat shorter timeframe. Why do these views hold, in the face of reasoned criticisms? One reason is that the predominant view is among the reasonable hypotheses interpreting the large body of empirical data; another is the social influences described in Chapters 3 and 4. But this section argues that there is a third reason, which is that the ubiquitous reasoning patterns and commitments already discussed, along with more specific methodologies typical of the ADHD sciences, demand certain characteristics of scientifically useful concepts. These demands significantly influence—and sometimes constrain—the choice of viable models. The influences and constraints are more scientifically and clinically significant than is often appreciated, both shaping the concept into its current form and holding it in place.[10]

Biological Focus, Reductionism

The biological focus in ADHD research is not accidental. For purposes of demonstrating cross-field data convergence, interlevel causal linkages, and appropriately scaled generalizations; devising clear operationalizations; and identifying mechanisms, work in biological sciences readily contributes to the goals. Many of the same factors also favor reductionism—again, as a tendency, not a scientific absolute.

Physical Entities

The reasons for the close match begin with science's overarching commitment to dealing with physical entities. This starting point means that some levels of investigation are de-emphasized. Social circumstances, for example, might in principle be physical but are often too complex to characterize in purely physical terms. The concept of "the family," for example, involves intangibles such as people's "relationships." Psychological and behavioral levels often have similarly unclear physical underpinnings; as discussed above, constructs like intelligence and aggression are not easily parsed in purely physical terms. Science does not ignore cognitive, behavioral, relational, or social levels, as we have seen in discussions of interlevel explanation, but they are not the main focus of ADHD science as a whole.[11] Instead, the sciences of ADHD embed the neuroscientific assumption that all behavior and mental states have a physical—that is, biological—basis. This assumption takes into account that the biological bases of cognition, emotion, and behavior respond to environmental factors. Yet it suggests that causal chains explaining these (and other) levels remain incomplete until the biological underpinnings are understood. If, in addition, complete explanations or progress toward them are indeed the research goal, then neuroscientific research will tend toward biological levels overall, if not within a single study or discipline; this tendency is a feature of *reduction*, which is explained in the next section.

Mechanism

The goal of demonstrating mechanisms favors a biological focus for similar reasons. Research at nonbiological (or not-only-biological or not-necessarily-biological) levels, such as sociological or educational research, can typically derive *correlations* among phenomena, but it cannot detail the processes underlying the correlations. Typically in the clinical sciences, the goal of demonstrating mechanisms is both biological and *reductive*—the science seeks to describe increasingly fundamental and detailed mechanisms for phenomena.

A consequence of the focus on mechanism that concerns some critics is the potential to downplay the "big picture"—context that might be observed by studying social systems, human interactions, long-term life experiences, and other phenomena not easily reducible to detailed mechanisms. In downplaying these levels of analysis, the argument goes, the focus on mechanism tends to miss out on factors that are simply not observable from a low-level point of view. For example, the higher-level role of classroom structure and requirements in ADHD symptomatology might be overlooked in the search for mechanisms of dopamine function. This criticism singles out *reductionism*—favoring reductive analysis to the detriment of other important perspectives.

Bechtel argues that the goal of detailing mechanisms, far from being reductive,[12] is inherently interlevel (Bechtel, 2008). He agrees that one ultimate goal of mechanistic analysis of biological phenomena is to demonstrate the details of finer and finer parts, and that the goal is in that sense reductive. But he emphasizes that understanding the detail can only be one goal. The mechanism and its parts are also organized within a larger system, and the organization is crucial to the mechanism's function. The mechanism contributes something to the larger system by performing an operation on some aspect of its environment, and the mechanism is facilitated or constrained by factors in its environment. A mechanistic explanation of a phenomenon of necessity must, then, be interlevel, including the mechanism of interest, its (lower-level) parts, and the (higher-level) wider environment in which the mechanism is situated.

Bechtel argues further that sciences that are not as concerned with interlevel "mechanistically mediated effects" but, rather, with causation (or, I would add, correlation) at the same level can retain their usefulness and their unique vocabularies. If we envision the goal of mechanistic explanation being vertical (digging deeper), the not-so-mechanistically inclined sciences look horizontally. To study respiration in amphibians, mechanistically inclined scientists might focus on the details of oxygen metabolism, while the scientist interested in higher levels might study shifting oxygen levels in a newt's or frog's environment. Both perspectives contribute to the goal. Applied to the sciences of ADHD, some researchers might study the details of neurotransmitter contributions to a measure of attention; scientists in a higher-level field could study how variations in education strategy contribute to attention to schoolwork—in the future, the relevance of each to the other might be as clear as it is in the respiration case. We have already seen such attempts being made in the interlevel theory proposed by Sagvolden. Other biologically oriented researchers, too, propose such theories, or at least frame their investigations in the higher-level context of its relevance to ADHD (itself a concept defined in higher-level behavioral and psychological terms).

Bechtel's argument is thus convincing that search for mechanisms, although reductive in strategy, is not *inherently* reductionistic in the sense that concerns critics. In practice, too, many scientists propose interlevel explanations and contextualize their findings. But those efforts are not the same as a goal of *finding out more about the context*. Although some descriptive research does study the "big picture" (the view of interest to higher-level scientists), in the case of ADHD science, these views have received less attention. It is probably undecidable whether this results more from a trick of funding or from a predominant scientific drive to reductively explore mechanism. In the former case, the goal of finding out more about context (environmental triggers, classroom effects, social attitudes, etc.) can be addressed simply by providing funding for such work. In the latter case, as long as the higher levels are thought of as "context," while the lower levels contribute to (real, true) "explanation," reductive research will dominate. In this circumstance, scientific goals reinforce viewing ADHD as a biological phenomenon, situated within individuals.

Tractability, Pragmatics

Practical considerations often favor biological models. Controlled study of individuals' biology is difficult, but it is relatively more manageable than controlled study of epidemiological, social, or relational phenomena, where the number of variables increases and the ability to control them decreases. It is also simpler to clarify and agree on operationalizations at the biological level. Defining "increased activity in the mesolimbic system" is relatively straightforward, given an average activity in the mesolimbic system as measured by a chosen procedure. Operationalizing a higher-level phenonmenon like "aggression," however, can be extremely contentious: Does one include only physical violence? Threatening behavior? Verbal subterfuge? One person's "aggression" can be another's favored behavior.[13] Finally, the availability of model organisms also makes biological work more tractable, decreasing the ethical dilemmas and requirements, as well as the expense, of working with human subjects.[14]

Science's requirement for experimental tractability also favors reductionism. The tighter experimental control possible at lower levels simplifies data interpretation, often making a given conclusion more convincing than one concerning higher levels. Finally, social factors can pragmatically encourage reductionism. Patterns of research funding, such as the NIH's "decade of the brain" and the pharmaceutical industry's funding of basic as well as neurologically oriented clinical research are cases in point. These factors are discussed in detail in Chapters 3 and 4.

Clinical Focus

Because ADHD is a medical (or medicalized) condition, research predominantly focuses on the models that work within the framework of medical needs. As discussed in Chapter 1, medicine's sphere of influence is with individuals, and primarily with aspects of human biology; drug treatment is medicine's chief contribution to ADHD management. In keeping with this, the quantity of research on pharmaceutical interventions overwhelms the quantity on behavioral or academic interventions (*see* data, Chapter 4). Similarly, the search for identifiable neurophysiological differences suits medical needs, as these differences may someday contribute to diagnosis. Reductionism driven by medical needs is always in tension with antireductionist needs of "the whole person." Still, clinical needs encourage narrowing of scientific focus to pharmacological solutions, given their relative efficiency by certain criteria; again, this phenomenon is discussed more fully in Chapter 4.

Dichotomization and Accumulated Difference

Although medicine and science typically depict ADHD as a property of individuals, the individuals are understood as being relatively (and relevantly) homogeneous. In medicine, although uniqueness is recognized, routines of diagnosis and treatment downplay individual variation. In science, common methodologies and statistical analyses do the same. As with the focus on biology, the end result—the homogenization and dichotomization of an "ADHD" type (with subtypes)—is a trend, rather than a necessity. Routine processes of categorizing, generalizing, and measuring and reporting on group averages, however, strengthen the trend. Together with the tendency to stick to traveled research paths, these processes allow differences to accumulate, further strengthening the end result.

Generalization

Creating a category entails generalizing about its members. But even for very simple entities, such as atoms or molecules, generalizations are inexact: some molecules in a sample of seemingly pure water (H_2O) will turn out to be deuterted water (DHO). In complex systems or organisms, the variability becomes more extensive and often more problematic. Birdwatchers are familiar with this difficulty: the illustrations in the field guide suggest that birds come in invariant types, but individual birds often fail to match the pictures. Nevertheless, for the purposes of categorizing, group members—water molecules, blue-winged warblers, ADHD diagnosed people—are lumped as though they were relevantly similar—which they often are, but not invariantly.[15] Further generalizations are then made about the general categories: "Arctic terns," on average, migrate 22,000 miles annually. "ADHD patients," on average, "have structural abnormalities of the cerebellum (Bush, 2010, 286)." These generalizations, along with many others, become part of reasoning chains that employ convergence and interlevel linkages. Throughout, the process of generalizing tends to homogenize variability.

In addition, scientific interest in generalizations, along with many statistical methodologies (*see* below) places questions about specific individuals beyond its purview. Questions such as "does this generalization apply to me?," "why me?," or "how me?" cannot be answered by current science (even with modern genomics), given individual uniqueness and methodological limitations.[16] The relative unapproachability of studying individuals, and the concomitant disinterest in variation as opposed to the typical, again serves to structure a relatively homogenized view of ADHD.

Averages

Determining an average value for some measured feature of interest is a more specific process than that of generalizing about a category; it is the basis of many common methodologies in scientific research. The researcher typically goes on to compare the average values of two or more groups, or the average values of a single group before and after an intervention. For example, Bush points out that "Functional and structural imaging studies generally use group-averaging and between-group statistical analyses, owing to the usually limited power to detect differences in individuals (Bush, 2010, 285)." Similarly, a scientist might compare "ADHD" and "control" (non-ADHD) groups on their average accuracy on a test of attention; or s/he might compare the average accuracy of the "ADHD" group before taking a medication with the group's average accuracy after taking a medication. In reporting the average, the researchers commonly (not always) bypass interpretation of individual data points or reasons for the spread or variability in the data. When this is the case, the averages elide intra-group differences among study subjects. If researchers then interpret the averages as representative of a group—which they typically do—another aspect of scientific practice reinforces a homogenized view of ADHD.

Countervailing tendencies might seem to protect against homogenization. ADHD-diagnosable individuals are clearly dissimilar with respect to the traits and behaviors often studied. The disjunctive diagnostic strategy of the DSM, in which symptoms are selected from a menu,[17] allows many different behavior patterns to be diagnosable as ADHD. In addition, many scientists recognize other reasons to expect that ADHD-diagnosable individuals are dissimilar. ADHD's multiple and variable comorbidities, great range in severity, and lack of a clear genomic pattern all suggest the possibility that intra-group differences might be important. For these reasons, researchers do design studies that allow finer-grained interpretations, choosing subjects according to subgroups such as ADHD subtype, ADHD severity, gender, age, or comorbidity profile. However, this is often not done, and, to the extent that researchers do not tease out heterogeneities, the result is a misleading nonambiguity in scientific findings.[18]

A study by Durston et al. provides an interesting example (Durston, et al., 2004). Durston et al. measured cerebral and intracranial volumes in ADHD-affected boys, their unaffected siblings, and normal controls (there were 30 boys in each group) using MRI. They reported that patients had significantly smaller intracranial volumes than controls (intracranial volume is a proxy for brain size); siblings and patients did not differ significantly, nor did control and sibling. The authors conclude that the ADHD-affected boys have a statistically significant 4.0% reduction in intracranial volume, and that this reduction reflects the biological basis of ADHD. But the measured differences are small, and the overlap between groups is almost complete. Thus, the conclusion that "a 4.0% reduction in intracranial volume was found in subjects with ADHD..." (332) is substantiated as long as subjects are considered as a group. Thinking of ADHD-diagnosed people as individuals, however, it is clear that the claim cannot be made with certainty about any particular ADHD-diagnosed child. That is, there is no guarantee that the child fits the "type" by the criterion being established in the article: the child was chosen as an "ADHD" subject because of behavioral fit with the behavioral criteria, but he may not have "smaller intracranial volume" than a child in the control group. Durston et al. make it clear that this is the case: they specify that if an ADHD-diagnosed child were to have an MRI, there is not enough knowledge of intracranial or cerebral size parameters to assess whether s/he has a deficit. Still, their conclusion about "subjects with ADHD" elides information about the details of their data, and reinforces a typological view of ADHD.

Dichotomization

Generalizations are clearer if they concern well demarcated categories, favoring definitions that meet this standard. The DSM's categorical approach to diagnosis attempts clear categorization—ADHD vs. other mental disorders; ADHD vs. "normal"— supporting the purposes of scientific practice. Typical methodology in the clinical sciences also supports the categorical view.

Clinical scientists commonly compare a group of individuals they determine to be affected by a condition of interest with another not so affected. In the case of ADHD, the resulting groups are most often the "ADHD" (sometimes differentiated further by subtype, comorbidity, gender, or other parameters) and "control" groups.[19] The division into groups assumes that the group members are distinct enough to be reliably recognized, and that the differences that make them distinctive correspond reliably with the division of interest, such as the ADHD-diagnosable/non-diagnosable division. This is problematic in the case of ADHD because of the marked fuzziness of the diagnostic boundary. That is not the main point that is important in this context, however. More significant is the joint effect of a tendency in methodology and an assumption. The methodological tendency is that researchers divide subjects into groups primarily for the purpose of observing *differences*, rather than similarities, between groups. The assumption is that the distinguishing differences between groups, and the correlates sought in the research, are *important* enough to be worth repeated classification and study. The focus on "important differences" de-emphasizes similarities between ADHD-diagnosable and non-diagnosable individuals, and contributes to dichotomization.

Thus, common methodologies reinforce the idea that "ADHD" and "normal" are distinct human types, despite the extensive overlap scientists acknowledge. This dichotomization into human types reinforces DSM-defined models of ADHD, particularly the DSM's categorical conception of classification.

Stasis

Together, then, the needs, commitments, and common methodologies of science have shaped core aspects of the current view of ADHD. They have contributed to (1) a biological focus, and to a tendency to reductionism; and (2) via generalizations and averaging, and via emphasis on certain methodologies, to a sharpening of between-groups differences and homogenization of within-groups differences that favor categorical models that dichotomize ADHD from "normal."

Other aspects of scientific practice contribute to the *continuation* of a particular concept rather than to the *structure* of the concept. ADHD and its historical precursors (see Chapter 1) have been studied since the 1960s—intensively since the 1980s. Intrascientific objections to the construct's validity have been available throughout that period, but they are only recently (25 to 30 years into intensive study) gaining traction, and the DSM-5's revisions are unlikely to encourage major change (*see* Chapter 6 for detail). This resistance to theory change is relative, and not immune to disruption (below, I discuss research that is beginning to change views of ADHD).[20] Yet the effect is strong, particularly when reinforced by other circumstances, such as the values and interests discussed in Chapters 3 through 5.

A distinction is central to the point of this section: It is one thing for scientists to continue to assume a concept or model for practical reasons, knowing that it is temporary, inadequate, or otherwise uncertain; it is another for scientists to continue to assume a concept or model in the belief that it is (approximately) true, correct, empirically adequate, or otherwise "on the right track." In the former case, the endorsement of the model is pragmatic; in the latter it is epistemic. This distinction is not sharp—scientists (like the rest of us) adopt different degrees and mixtures of epistemic and pragmatic endorsement. As a whole, though, the ADHD literature does not question the direction of the research, put the term "ADHD" in scare quotes, comment on future models, or otherwise give indication that the predominant view of ADHD is merely pragmatic. Thus, although it is true that scientific practice gives researchers strong pragmatic reasons to decide on a model and stick with it,[21] it is also the case that scientific practice—apart from empirical data—reinforces the epistemic endorsement that is evident in scientific literature and practice. How so?

Traveled Paths

The goal of demonstrating data convergence and interlevel causal links relies on previous work; the reasoner's inferences rightly converge with or link to prior categories only if her/his operationalizations and other categories match the earlier ones. This circumstance encourages modeling and inquiry along traveled paths. For example, look again at Sagvolden et al.'s argument linking data on the neurophysiology of dopamine to parenting styles and cultural expectations (*see* p. 51). Multiple categories of objects, people, and other phenomena are needed for this argument: neurotransmitters, neuroanatomical structures, reinforcement schedules, rats and humans, rat and human behavior, parents and parenting skills, and cultures and cultural expectations. Which categories are available and what links intelligible depend in large part on categories and links established by previous efforts. Similarly, thinking in terms of methods and experimental practice rather than theory, experimentation needs to work with accepted tools, techniques, and experimental models to replicate results. This is one way to say that science builds on previous science; but it is also to say that previous science constrains current science to some extent—novelty is not forbidden, just difficult—by imposing a structure of prior formulations, categorizations, and contexts—and tools, techniques, and experimental models—of interest.[22]

The most central of the favored categories is that of "ADHD" itself. Despite the range of unknowns, most basic science and clinical ADHD research has in common that it presupposes DSM-defined ADHD rather than investigating ADHD-correlated phenomena independent of that model. (Murphy [2006] notes this phenomenon generally for psychiatric research.) Scientists choose research subjects because they exhibit DSM-defined symptoms, contrast them with "controls," and interpret data relative to that distinction. In doing so, researchers have, over several decades, documented myriad statistically significant differences between those who are ADHD-diagnosable and those who are not. The positive results buttress the epistemic (as opposed to pragmatic) reasons to retain the category. This effect, however, is exaggerated by the pragmatically based practice of sticking with "ADHD."

Accumulated Differences

As discussed above, researchers can in principle find either differences or similarities between groups they compare. Typically, though, a study's methodology focuses on finding differences, and a "positive"—and therefore more likely to be published—study is one that does so. The differences, cumulatively, contribute to a set of correlates with the phenomenon being investigated. ADHD correlates include various socially disvalued differences from "normal," such as lower income (Birnbaum et al., 2005), increased incidence of substance abuse (Wilens, Faraone, Biederman, & Gunawardene, 2003), and "poorer" scores on tests of attention (Dimoska et al., 2003), along with a multiplicity of physiological differences. Correlations like these have, to date, reinforced the predominant view of ADHD as a biological dysfunction.

One interpretation of this is, simply, that the current concept, although needing refinement, is on the right track. That is, the concept has been adopted because it is approximately correct, not because it is scientifically tractable or because it fits medical, scientific, or social needs or preconceptions. However, the problem with the emphasis on difference-finding is that when one seeks differences one can often find them—that does not mean that the differences are necessarily important,or that there aren't alternative ways of studying a phenomenon that might yield more important differences (or similarities). Scientists know this in principle, of course. But the prevailing impetus is such that alternative interpretations tend to be downplayed. To take an egregious example, Barkley et al. (1993) undertook a survey to assess the correlation between risky driving behaviors/accidents and ADHD diagnosis in adolescents and young adults. The authors concluded that ADHD and increased driving risks were associated—but the cited results suggest that ADHD is not necessary to explain the poorer driving ratings of the subjects. Except for driving without a license, all the surveyed outcomes, including license revocation, motor vehicle crashes, crash-related injuries, and number of traffic citations, also correlate highly with comorbid oppositional defiant disorder (ODD).[23] Although the authors specify that "...ratings of ADHD are highly correlated with those of ODD in these samples ($r = .91$)...making it unclear as to which is most important in the relationship to the outcomes...(217)," they nevertheless conclude, one sentence later, that "[i]ndividuals with ADHD followed into late adolescence and young adulthood have a significantly greater risk as drivers than normal control subjects (217)." The conclusion section of the article's abstract is only slightly more guarded about making this move, reading, "ADHD, and especially its association with oppositional defiant disorder/conduct disorder, is associated with substantially increased risks for driving...(212)." Thus, a result that seems to be largely confined to the subset of ADHD-diagnosable individuals who also have ODD, or perhaps simply to young people who have ODD, is attributed to ADHD per se. By interpreting their data relative to ADHD (and not to the salient alternative, ODD), the authors' conclusion reflects *that choice* as much it reflects the data.

A contrast may make the effect clearer. Woodward et al. (2000) take possibilities other than DSM-defined ADHD into account in understanding driving outcomes in young people. Their study attempted to discover what the role of "attentional difficulties" (not ADHD according to the medical/DSM model) might be on driving records, but they also considered possible effects of family function, social background, gender, and conduct problems. These alternatives explained 10 of 11 driving-risk-related behaviors and outcomes, the single exception being the risk of a motor vehicle accident involving injury. Interestingly, even in this study, relative emphasis is placed on that remaining correlation with attentional difficulties. However, in interpreting the data relative to alternatives, rather than to DSM-defined ADHD, the authors demonstrate that social and familial factors, rather than a diagnosis, may[24] go a long way toward explaining diagnosable adolescents' poor driving records. Such conclusions do not contribute to the accumulating differences between ADHD-diagnosable and non-diagnosable people. Rather, they implicitly question whether that distinction is the important one in the case being investigated.

Another way the emphasis on accumulating differences reveals itself is that even when the data indicate "*no* significant difference," researchers often interpret the result as a need for future, more refined diagnostic tests (Durston et al., 2004) or means of intervention (Jensen et al., 2007). That is, the expectation is held out that there probably *is* a difference, because that is what the ADHD model predicts; it simply cannot be detected with present means of testing or intervention.[25] In this way, sticking with the current ADHD model leads to de-emphasizing the relevant alternative that there might be no significant difference in the measure in question.

Complicating Categories?

A contravening tendency does exist, however—some scientists *do* undertake alternative strategies, recognizing complications, exceptions, inconsistent results, and other difficulties with the predominant view of ADHD. ADHD experts are beginning to address, as well, the clinically important issues of ADHD's heterogeneity, comorbidities, variable expression within individuals, and fuzzy boundaries. For example, they identify and study ADHD endophenotypes (Castellanos et al., 2009),[26] traits or behaviors that cross diagnostic categories (anxiety, restlessness), and alternative animal models. Recent neurocircuitry models suggest that deficits might disrupt complexly interacting systems, imbalancing brain function in variable ways—alternatives to models proposing single or isolated deficits intended to explain the range of symptoms (Bush, 2010).[27] Finer-grained analyses are proceeding in work on the genetics of ADHD as well. Molecular geneticists (and others) have associated candidate genes[28] with the function of the neurotransmitters dopamine, norepinephrine, serotonin, and acetylcholine, and with neural development, neural plasticity, and reward systems (Gizer et al., 2009). Although none of the candidates has yet been strongly associated with ADHD or an ADHD subtype, ADHD's heterogeneity may explain this. Given these and other attempts, it may be that science is on the cusp of a new concept or set of concepts that will more clearly describe and explain ADHD, in all its heterogeneity.

Yet many alternatives remain little studied. With respect to ADHD's etiology, for example, many genetic and neuroimaging studies have been done. Many-fold fewer, however, seek environmental triggers or gene–environment interactions. Similarly, although there has long been interest in studying interventions other than medication, and many alternatives continue to be explored, the relative number of studies remains greatly slanted toward pharmacotherapy (*see* Chapter 4 for details).

Thus, the tendencies toward stasis do not represent tight constraints. Presumably, if new studies produced too few results consistent with the DSM-defined construct, or if anomalies became salient enough, there would be an irresistible impetus for change. Presently, however, although it is true that (1) the field of ADHD research is active, with multiple, competing hypotheses in play; (2) scientists consider alternatives models, some of which do not line up with the present conceptions of ADHD; and (3) hypotheses in which heterogeneity and variability are expressly recognized have potential to break down the existing homogenization of the categories, the balance still leans toward stasis. Researchers continue to find small differences between standardly defined "control" and "affected" groups, and to deem those differences important. In this way—even as new models are proposed—repeated mining of the ADHD/control difference decreases the perceived need to consider new models, while reinforcing epistemic reasons to support the predominant one. Finally, and very powerfully, social circumstances contribute to maintaining the prevailing concept; these are discussed in Chapters 3 and 4. At least as I write in 2013, the predominant view of ADHD persists. In substance, if not in detail, it is likely to continue to do so for some time: Changes in the DSM-5 refine and expand but do not overhaul the ADHD category (Hawthorne, 2010; *see* Chapter 6).

Reification

In the questions science addresses, the reasoning patterns and methodologies employed in addressing the questions, and in setting some issues aside, science structures the conception of ADHD along particular lines. These practices also contribute to another aspect of stasis: the *reification* of an ADHD type. DSM-defined ADHD has been used in thousands of studies in hundreds of journals. The more the scientific practices detailed in this section reinforce the existing model, the more natural thinking in terms of the differences it implies becomes. Many individual scientists likely do think of ADHD as a heuristic or as provisional. Yet both subject selection methodology and the emphasis on the scientific work's clinical significance—as expressed in concluding comments of research papers, for example—suggest that the ADHD construct is intended to designate an identifiable, treatable—hence reified—kind (with three subtypes), not just to serve as a device for thinking about people or behaviors. Consider the oddity, for example, of repeatedly dividing one's research subjects into "ADHD" and "control" groups without simultaneously thinking that there is—*really*—a difference between the individuals in the groups.

It is true that in some ways, the identification and reification of an ADHD category is little different than any other definition or classification scientists do—of molecules, rocks, bacteria, birds, ecological niches, economic strata, etc. But, of course, the ADHD category changes the lives of those to whom it is applied, and it alters the wider social world as well (*see* Chapter 5). Understanding where the ADHD category comes from—and the extent to which it is optional—can give important reasons to accept or question it.

Conclusion

Progress in the neurosciences makes predicting the future of ADHD sciences uncertain. New methods, new foci, and new ways of considering data may develop alongside expanding empirical observations. At present, however, the patterns picked out here apply much more broadly. Scientists studying other mental disorders employ similar reasoning strategies and methodologies, so that controversial degrees of biological focus, reduction, homogenization, dichotomization, and reification affect research on depression, substance abuse, personality disorders—even study of more deeply impairing disorders such as autism and schizophrenia.[29] Other fields, too, employ categories influenced by the needs and commitments of science.

However, the effects described in this chapter do not work in isolation. The tendencies that affect the sciences of ADHD do so in part because the study of science is not an isolated phenomenon. Scientists are people, members of a society. Their work is supported and influenced by socially available concepts—and funding, of course. In the clinical sciences, the mutual influences of medicine on science and science on medicine are continuous. And the mutual influences of the wider society on science and science on wider society are continuous as well. For this reason, I re-emphasize that the current concept of ADHD has been *jointly* determined by science, medicine, and the wider society, each playing roles that can only partly be disentangled. Chapter 3 describes the role of the wider society.

REFERENCES

American Psychiatric Association (2000). *Diagnostic and Statistical Manual of Mental Disorders* (4, Text Revision ed.). Arlington, VA: American Psychiatric Association.

American Psychiatric Association (2013). *Diagnostic and Statistical Manual of Mental Disorders: DSM-5* (5th ed.). Washington, DC: American Psychiatric Association.

Anhalt, K., McNeil, C. B., & Bahl, A. B. (1998). The ADHD classroom kit: a whole-classroom approach for managing disruptive behavior. *Psychology in the Schools, 35*(1), 67–79.

Barkley, R. A., Guevremont, D. C., Anastopoulos, A. D., DuPaul, G. J., & Shelton, T. L. (1993). Driving-related risks and outcomes of attention deficit hyperactivity disorder in adolescents and young adults: a 3- to 5-year follow-up survey. *Pediatrics, 92*(2), 212–218.

Barry, T. D., Lyman, R. D., & Klinger, L. G. (2002). Academic underachievement and attention-deficit/hyperactivity disorder: the negative impact of symptom severity on school performance. *Journal of School Psychology, 40*(3), 259–283.

Beatty, J. (1995). The evolutionary contingency thesis. In G. Wolters & J. G. Lennox (Eds.), *Concepts, Theories, and Rationality in the Biological Sciences: The Second Pittsburgh-Konstanz Colloquium in the Philosophy of Science, University of Pittsburgh, October 1–4, 1993* (pp. 45–82). Pittsburgh, PA: University of Pittsburgh Press.

Bechtel, W. (2008). *Mental Mechanisms: Philosophical Perspectives on Cognitive Neuroscience.* New York: Taylor and Francis.

Birnbaum, H. G., Kessler, R. C., Lowe, S. W., Secnik, K., Greenberg, P. E., Leong, S. A., et al. (2005). Costs of attention-deficit hyperactivity disorder (ADHD) in the US: Excess costs of persons with ADHD and their family members in 2000. *Current Medical Research and Opinion, 21*(2), 195–206.

Braaten, E. B., Beiderman, J., Monuteaux, M. C., Mick, E., Calhoun, E., Cattan, G., et al. (2003). Revisiting the association between attention-deficit/hyperactivity disorder and anxiety disorders: a familial risk analysis. *Biol Psychiatry, 53*(1), 93–99.

Bush, G. (2010). Attention-deficit/hyperactivity disorder and attention networks. *Neuropsychopharmacology, 35*(1), 278–300.

Castellanos, F. X., Kelly, C., & Milham, M. P. (2009). The restless brain: Attention-deficit hyperactivity disorder, resting-state functional connectivity, and intrasubject variability. *The Canadian Journal of Psychiatry, 54*(10), 665–672.

Christakis, D. A., Zimmerman, F. J., DiGiuseppe, D. L., & McCarty, C. A. (2004). Early television exposure and subsequent attentional problems in children. *Pediatrics, 113*(4), 708–713.

Coghill, D., Nigg, J., Rothenberger, A., Sonuga-Barke, E., & Tannock, R. (2005). Whither causal models in the neuroscience of ADHD? *Developmental Science, 8*(2), 105–114.

Darden, L., & Craver, C. (2002). Strategies in the interfield discovery of the mechanism of protein synthesis. *Studies in History and Philosophy of Biological and Biomedical Sciences, 33*, 1–28.

Dimoska, A., Johnstone, S. J., Barry, R. J., & Clarke, A. R. (2003). Inhibitory motor control in children with attention-deficit/hyperactivity disorder: event-related potentials in the stop-signal paradigm. *Biological Psychiatry, 54*, 1345–1354.

Dopheide, J. A., & Pliszka, S. R. (2009). Reviews of therapeutics: Attention-deficit—hyperactivity disorder: an update. *Pharmacotherapy, 29*(6), 656–679.

Dumit, J. (2004). *Picturing Personhood: Brain Scans and Biomedical Identity*. Princeton, NJ: Princeton University Press.

Durston, S. (2008). Converging methods in studying attention-deficit/hyperactivity disorder: what can we learn from neuroimaging and genetics? *Development and Psychopathology, 20*, 1133–1143.

Durston, S., Pol, H. E. H., Schnack, H. G., Buitelaar, J. K., Steenhuis, M. P., Minderaa, R. B., et al. (2004). Magnetic resonance imaging of boys with attention-deficit/hyperactivity disorder and their unaffected siblings. *Journal of the American Academy of Child and Adolescent Psychiatry, 43*(3), 332–340.

Durston, S., Tottenham, N. T., Thomas, K. M., Davidson, M. C., Eigsti, I.-M., Yang, Y., et al. (2003). Differential patterns of striatal activation in young children with and without ADHD. *Biological Psychiatry, 53*, 871–878.

Franke, B., Neale, B. M., & Faraone, S. V. (2009). Genome-wide association studies in ADHD. *Hum Genet, 126*(1), 13–50.

Gizer, I. R., Ficks, C., & Waldman, I. D. (2009). Candidate gene studies of ADHD: a meta-analytic review. *Human Genetics, 126*, 51–90.

Glennan, S. (2002). Rethinking mechanistic explanation. *Philosophy of Science, 69*(Supplement), S342–S353.

Haack, S. (1995). Puzzling out science. *Academic Questions, 8*(2), 20–31.

Haslam, N., Williams, B., Prior, M., Haslam, R., Graetz, B., & Sawyer, M. (2006). The latent structure of attention-deficit/hyperactivity disorder: a taxometric analysis. *Australian and New Zealand Journal of Psychiatry, 40*, 639–647.

Hawthorne, S. (2010). Redefining ADHD: Disagreement Over Values. *Bioethics Forum*. Retrieved January 14, 2011, from http://www.thehastingscenter.org/

Bioethicsforum/Post.aspx?id=4615&blogid=140&terms=hawthorne+and+%23filename+*.html

Heinrich, H., Gevensleben, H., Freislander, F. J., Moll, G. H., & Rothenberger, A. (2004). Training of slow cortical potentials in attention-deficit/hyperactivity disorder: evidence for positive behavioral and neurophysiological effects. *Biological Psychiatry, 55,* 772–775.

Jensen, P. S., Arnold, L. E., Swanson, J. M., Vitiello, B., Abikoff, H. B., Greenhill, L. L., et al. (2007). 3-year follow-up of the NIMH MTA study. *Journal of the American Academy of Child and Adolescent Psychiatry, 46*(8), 989–1002.

Jensen, P. S., Garcia, J. A., Glied, S., Crowe, M., Foster, M., Schlander, M., et al. (2005). Cost-effectiveness of ADHD treatments: Findings from the Multimodal Treatment Study of Children with ADHD. *American Journal of Psychiatry, 162*(9), 1628–1636.

Karatekin, C. (2005). A comprehensive and developmental theory of ADHD is tantalizing, but premature. *Behavioral and Brain Sciences, 28*(3), 430–431.

Kuhn, T. S. (1996 [1962]). *The Structure of Scientific Revolutions* (3 ed.). Chicago: University of Chicago Press.

Longino, H. E. (2001). What do we measure when we measure aggression? *Studies in the History and Philosophy of Science, 32*(4), 685–704.

Machamer, P., Darden, L., & Craver, C. F. (2000). Thinking about mechanisms. *Philosophy of Science, 67*(1), 1–25.

Mayes, R., Bagwell, C., & Erkulwater, J. (2009). *Medicating Children: ADHD and Pediatric Mental Health.* Cambridge, MA: Harvard University Press.

Mayes, S. D., Calhoun, S. L., & Crowell, E. W. (2000). Learning disabilities and ADHD: Overlapping spectrum disorders. *Journal of Learning Disabilities, 33*(5), 417–424.

Miranda, A., & Presentacion, M. J. (2000). Efficacy of cognitive-behavioral therapy in the treatment of children with ADHD, with and without aggressiveness. *Psychology in the Schools, 37*(2), 169–182.

Murphy, D. (2006). *Psychiatry in the Scientific Image.* Cambridge, MA: The MIT Press.

Ohan, J. L., & Johnston, C. (2007). What is the social impact of ADHD in girls? A multi-method assessment. *J Abnorm Child Psychol, 35*(2), 239–250.

Ostrander, R., Crystal, D. S., & August, G. (2006). Attention deficit-hyperactivity disorder, depression, and self- and other-assessments of social competence: a developmental study. *Journal of Abnormal Child Psychology, 34,* 773–787.

Parens, E., & Johnston, J. (2009). Facts, values, and Attention-Deficit Hyperactivity Disorder (ADHD): an update on the controversies. *Child Adolesc Psychiatry Ment Health, 3*(1), 1.

Pelham, W. E., & Fabiano, G. A. (2008). Evidence-based psychosocial treatments for attention-deficit/hyperactivity disorder. *Journal of Clinical Child and Adolescent Psychology, 37*(1), 184–214.

Rubia, K. (2005). RED: ADHD under the "micro-scope" of the rat model. *Behavioral and Brain Sciences*, *28*(3), 439–440.

Sagvolden, T., Aase, H., Johansen, E. B., & Russell, V. A. (2005). A dynamic developmental theory of attention-deficit/hyperactivity disorder (ADHD) predominantly hyperactive/impulsive and combined subtypes. *Behavioral and Brain Sciences*, *28*(3), 397–468.

Sagvolden, T., Johansen, E. B., Woien, G., Walaas, S. I., Storm-Mathisen, J., Bergersen, L. H., et al. (2009). The spontaneously hypertensive rat model of ADHD—the importance of selecting the appropriate reference strain. *Neuropharmacology*, *57*(7–8), 619–626.

Satterfield, J. H., & Schell, A. (1997). A prospective study of hyperactive boys with conduct problems and normal boys: adolescent and adult criminality. *Journal of the American Academy of Child and Adolescent Psychiatry*, *36*(12), 1726–1735.

Schaffner, K. F. (1993). *Discovery and Explanation in Biology and Medicine*. Chicago: The University of Chicago Press.

Shaw, P., Eckstrand, K., Sharp, W., Blumenthal, J., Lerch, J. P., Greenstein, D., et al. (2007). Attention-deficit/hyperactivity disorder is characterized by a delay in cortical maturation. *Proceedings of the National Academy of Science*, *104*(49), 19,649–19,654.

Singh, I. (2008). Beyond polemics: science and ethics of ADHD. *Nature Reviews: Neuroscience*, *9*, 957–964.

Sonuga-Barke, E. J. S., & Castellanos, F. X. (2005). A common core dysfunction in attention-deficit/hyperactivity disorder: A scientific red herring? *Behavioral and Brain Sciences*, *28*(3), 443–444.

Spencer, T. (2009). Toward a new understanding of attention-deficit hyperactivity disorder: advances in research and treatment. *CNS Drugs*, *23*(Suppl 1), 5–8.

Spencer, T., Biederman, J., Wilens, T., Faraone, S. V., Prince, J., Gerard, K., et al. (2001). Efficacy of a mixed amphetamine salts compound in adults with attention-deficit/hyperactivity disorder. *Archives of General Psychiatry*, *58*(8), 784–785.

Swing, E. L., Gentile, D. A., Anderson, C. A., & Walsh, D. A. (2010). Television and video game exposure and the development of attention problems. *Pediatrics*, *126*(2), 214–221.

Taylor, E. (2009). Developing ADHD. *The Journal of Child Psychology and Psychiatry*, *50*(1–2), 126–132.

Thagard, P. (1999). *How Scientists Explain Disease*. Princeton, NJ: Princeton University Press.

Tripp, G., & Wickens, J. R. (2009). Neurobiology of ADHD. *Neuropharmacology*, *57*(7–8), 579–589.

Wilens, T. E., Faraone, S. V., Biederman, J., & Gunawardene, S. (2003). Does stimulant therapy of attention-deficit/hyperactivity disorder beget later substance abuse? A meta-analytic review of the literature. *Pediatrics*, *111*(1), 179–185.

Woodruff, T. J., Axelrad, D. A., Kyle, A. D., Nweke, O., Miller, G. G., & Hurley, B. J. (2004). Trends in environmentally related childhood illnesses. *Pediatrics, 113*(4), 1133–1140.

Woodward, J. (2000). Explanation and invariance in the special sciences. *British Journal for the Philosophy of Science, 51,* 197–254.

Woodward, L. J., Fergusson, D. M., & Horwood, L. J. (2000). Driving outcomes of young people with attentional difficulties in adolescence. *Journal of the American Academy of Child and Adolescent Psychiatry, 39*(5), 627–634.

NOTES

1. I took the random sample from a search for articles having "ADHD" or "attention deficit hyperactivity disorder" or "attention deficit disorder" indexed in ERIC, PsychINFO, or PubMed and published between January 1, 1990 and June 13, 2009. I manually culled duplicates, anonymous articles, editorials, and literature reviews from the search results. If the sampled article concerned drug intervention, described ADHD's etiology as "neuronal" (or a similar term or concept), or measured biological parameters, I labeled the concept "biological." The biological majority is statistically significant by the Pearson Chi-square test. Additional details available on request.

2. Generalizations about a rare disease might have very narrow scope, applying to only a few individuals; in contrast, a generalization about DNA replication may apply to a broad scope of organisms. Likewise, some degree of invariance is necessary for a generalization to be useful; however, the degree needed changes according to the context. When stakes are high—for example, when the consequences of a mistake are bad—or when the science is more advanced, greater invariance must be demonstrated for a generalization to be acceptable. Lower stakes allow for generalizations with more exceptions (less invariance). Nevertheless, within parameters appropriate to a given interest, scientists prefer generalizations that have broader scope and greater invariance over those of lesser scope and lesser invariance.

3. The meaning and significance of "levels" in scientific explanation is a complexity I cannot delve into in detail. My usage is consistent with Bechtel's analysis (Bechtel, 2008), in which "levels" need to be understood locally: local in the ontological sense that the levels relevant to a given object of inquiry may not align in size or part–whole relations with those relevant to another object of inquiry, and local epistemologically as well, in varying with the goals and methodologies of various fields—particularly the broad divisions of physical science, biological science, behavioral/psychological science, and the humanities and social sciences.

4. Dozens of experts offered commentary on Sagvolden et al.'s hypothesis, many suggesting such alternatives (see *Behavior and Brain Sciences 2005; 28(3):419–450*).

5. Sagvolden et al. use a genetically mutant rat, the spontaneously hypertensive rat, to model ADHD because of presumed similarities in dopamine system dysfunction.
6. Reasoning by analogy is often considered intellectually suspect, given that it is neither deductive nor empirically demonstrative, but it can be demystified and defended. Paul Thagard provides a straightforward example that Joseph Lister used in formulating the germ theory of gangrene: (1) Fermentation is caused by germs; (2) Putrefaction (infection) following surgery is like fermentation. Therefore, putrefaction may be caused by germs (Thagard, 1999, 139). This basic analogical reasoning form—employing a premise of the form "X 'is like' Y"—is a commonplace in everyday reasoning, and in science as well. Simply recognizing the routine nature of the reasoning pattern helps to dispel some suspicion of it. Presumably, given its ubiquity and apparent usefulness, analogical reasoning *can* be sound. In addition, Thagard argues that analogy has heuristic benefits. It can transfer solutions known to work in one area to new problems, and it can improve explanations by linking one idea to another. Lister's analogy does both: It applies knowledge from Pasteur's work on fermentation to surgery, and it improves the explanation of putrefaction by a suggestion of convergence with the germ theory already applied in fermentation. Thagard suggests that animal models can be improved by assuring that causal processes in the animal model and in people are demonstrably and closely similar, as opposed to sharing superficial similarities. Use of multiple analogous systems (for example, demonstration of a phenomenon in both rats and nonhuman primates) can also, he says, improve such reasoning.
7. The boundary between descriptive and mechanistic studies is not sharp. If a scientist demonstrates that dose X of drug Y is consistently correlated with reaction Q, she may be justified in saying that the observation is not *mere* description, but, given other data, points toward a mechanism of action. Further study could give more detail of how drug Y works. Say the researcher finds that it permeates the blood–brain barrier at rate Z. We could say that this is not merely a description of penetration rate, but part of a mechanism. Still, our scientist can ask again how it penetrates the blood–brain barrier. This detailing process can continue through however many iterations are needed to satisfy the goals and/or capabilities of the scientist(s).
8. Some definitions of mechanism emphasize the "parts": Thagard, for example, defines mechanism as "...a system of parts that operate or interact like those of a machine, transmitting forces, motion, and energy to one another (Thagard, 1999, 106)." Glennan proposes, "A mechanism for a behavior is a complex system that produces that behavior by the interaction of a number of parts, where the interactions between parts can be characterized by direct, invariant, change-relating generalizations" (2002, S344). Others argue that the concept of mechanism includes both the parts (entities) and their actions (activities): mechanisms are "...entities and activities organized such that they are

productive of regular changes from start or set-up to finish or termination conditions (Machamer, Darden, & Craver, 2000, 3)." Each of these definitions is primarily linear (single-level), as opposed to Bechtel's expressly interlevel concept, although Machamer, Darden, and Craver argue that mechanisms in biology must be considered in context; in particular, they specify that entities and activities may have multiple roles at multiple levels. This contextualization, however, stops short of Bechtel's claim that the mechanisms are inherently interlevel.

9. Machamer, Darden, and Craver differentiate between a "mechanism schema" and a "mechanism sketch," the former being more complete. A "mechanism schema" specifies the entities and activities involved in a regular process of interest, although some details remain unclear; a "mechanism sketch" is a hypothesis in which some entities or activities remain unknown. Darden and Craver (2002) explain the process of filling in these details as "schema instantiation," "forward chaining" and "backtracking"—experimentation and theorizing that proposes and demonstrates the entities and activities needed to fill in gaps in understanding. Undertaking this process, they argue, requires that empirical observations or manipulations establish that phenomena observable at various levels or by various techniques are at least (1) consistently correlated with each other and, ideally, (2) that the correlation holds under manipulation of a relevant variable.

10. The nature and extent of the clinical significance is spelled out in Chapter 5.

11. More definitively ruled out are perspectives involving nonphysical interpretations of behavior, such as actions of immaterial souls.

12. Bechtel does not differentiate between science's methodologies being *reductive* and their being *reductionistic* in the senses I have defined in the text.

13. Longino discusses this example in detail in "What Do We Measure When We Measure Aggression?" (Longino, 2001).

14. Using animals in research *introduces* ethical dilemmas as well, but I will not take up this topic here.

15. Some differences, of course, are trivial relative to whatever the generalization is, but it may be hard to discern which are trivial and which are not.

16. This limitation of science is in tension with its clinical application to individuals; I explore some implications of this tension in Chapter 5.

17. Thank you to Helen Longino for this way of phrasing the point.

18. Even when studies are designed to detect differences in subgroups, the result may be additional problematic generalizations. See, for example, the discussion of research on ADHD and gender in Chapter 3.

19. Other comparisons include an ADHD group vs. a group diagnosed with another mental disorder, or two ADHD groups receiving and not receiving an intervention of interest.

20. Does ADHD science still count as young science with this timeframe? If so, one might object that the current level of questioning simply is a typical pace

for scientific change. I think there has already been adequate time to consider alternatives.
21. Many practical reasons center on communication. To study "ADHD," scientists need to study the syndrome described by the DSM model; if they study related or differently described phenomena, they risk making their work irrelevant to ADHD—hence to those who might otherwise have interest (academic, clinical, or for funding purposes) in their work. Sticking with the current model is efficient relative to the goal of learning more about ADHD as currently understood, and it allows comparisons between studies, as well as meta-analyses. ADHD, as an important clinical concern, also attracts research funding.
22. The phenomenon is more general than a Kuhnian paradigm (Kuhn, 1996 [1962])—the retained categories are at multiple levels and cross multiple fields; indeed, they are required for interdisciplinary work (unlike the Kuhnian notion of disciplinary isolation and incommensurability).
23. Oppositional defiant disorder, characterized by such behaviors as "often loses temper" and "often argues with adults" (American Psychiatric Association, 2000, 102) is at least as controversial a construct as ADHD, but discussion of the involved issues would go too far afield.
24. The "may" is important here because, as explained in the text, Woodward et al. did not select subjects according to DSM diagnosis.
25. Anthropologist Joseph Dumit observes a similar pattern in reasoning concerning planning and interpretation of positive emission tomography (PET) images of brains (Dumit, 2004, p. 68).
26. ADHD's endophenotypes are (or would be, if found) heritable differences that are consistently associated with particular presentations of ADHD.
27. Barkley's *dysfunctional behavioral inhibition model* and Sagvolden et al.'s *dynamic developmental theory* are single-deficit models. One neurocircuitry model is Sonuga-Barke and Castellanos' *default mode hypothesis,* in which dysfunctional interactions between activation of frontal brain areas and the brain's "downtime" activity—its default mode—lead to variability in response times on psychological tests, such as those measuring sustained attention, motor sequencing, time perception, and so forth. Sergeant proposes a *cognitive-energetic model,* in which there is dysfunctional interplay between top-down processes (executive function direction behavior) and bottom-up processes (Bush, 2010).
28. "Candidate genes" are genes that seem likely to be involved in ADHD etiology, given their function in the brain, the relation of that function to ADHD-associated behaviors, and demonstration that the genes are expressed (i.e., the proteins they "code for" are produced and active) in areas of the brain that are also linked to ADHD.
29. I would expect to find similar patterns in the study of some nonmental disorders or diseases as well.

3 SOCIAL ALLIES AND ADVERSARIES

In *The Pasteurization of France,* Bruno Latour retells the story of Louis Pasteur's discovery of the anthrax bacillus. Latour reframes the "discovery" as a reification, achieved not by isolated science but by Pasteur's work to forge alliances among scientists, farmers, hygienists, and even the anthrax bacillus.

After collecting soil samples from the French countryside, Pasteur and his colleagues did recognize a microscopic organism: it separated starch, grew on a specific culture medium, and had a characteristic appearance under a microscope. But to achieve this, Pasteur and his laboratory colleagues had to find ways to get the microbe to do what they needed: Pasteur's anthrax was an actant—an unwitting ally—interacting in the tale of its own "discovery." Pasteur defined the "anthrax bacillus" according to the scientists' actions *and its responses*. Once this step was completed, Pasteur took the formerly wild bacillus and a tamed vaccine derived from it back to the countryside. There, he dramatically demonstrated his success by infecting a flock of sheep with anthrax, preventing disease in half by inoculating them with the new vaccine. This demonstration recruited farmers as allies; their goal of saving their flocks aligned with Pasteur's of spreading his discovery. Pasteur also enlisted the French hygienists, who saw potential progress in their goal—preventing human disease—in Pasteur's results. In Latour's description, Pasteur quickly established a strong network and gained much funding for future research. Pasteur succeeded in "translating" old questions and terrors about epidemics into a model that allowed—or at least promised—control.[1]

A narrative about the discovery and popularization of ADHD can be similarly recast.[2] The now-reified ADHD concept helps solve the personal and social problems of multiple allies, among them those who are ADHD-diagnosable; their parents[3]; teachers and school administrators; scientists, physicians, and other healthcare providers; those who develop, manufacture, and sell ADHD medications or other treatment modalities for ADHD; and government officials who determine funding of ADHD research and frame rules for the various stakeholders. The personal and institutional values these and other individuals support and work toward help glue together an alliance that strongly supports DSM-defined ADHD. But this broad alliance did not simply grow up around a ready-made definition (or entity). Instead, just as the needs of medicine and science contribute to the structure of DSM-defined ADHD (*see* Chapters 1 and 2), the active "translation" (a Latourian concept I will make use of below) of ADHD by various constituencies has also shaped the predominant understanding. Simultaneously, institutional structures and practices, as well as some noninstitutionalized practices, come into adjustment with the category through reciprocal changes affecting social practices, medicine, and science.

The idea that ADHD is "constructed" in this way does not conflict with its addressing real problems. The issues faced by diagnosable individuals, the schools, parents, clinicians, and others and the relevance of individual neurophysiology to the difficulties faced—all of these are tangible phenomena. As in the medical and scientific views of ADHD, however, the social views might have been parsed differently, yet our society has decided on the current category. The first section of this chapter details some of the goals, interests, and ethical values the diagnostic category helps forward, along with ways it has been integrated into policy and practice in a number of social structures. In an ongoing process, social needs help shape the category, while the category encourages changes in society.

Despite their current strength, the social contributions are unstable. The second section of this chapter examines multiple controversies concerning the roles, tactics, and degrees of success of social institutions in defining and using the ADHD category. These fall under broad themes of mismatch among the various constituencies' goals and actual practice and results. Questions surround the efficacy of current models and treatments; the equity of practice, such as the unequal diagnosis and treatment rates among races and genders; worry about medicalization, including concern over the essentializing and labeling of individuals; and suspicions about manipulation of lay and medical understanding of the category by pharmaceutical companies.[4] Many of these controversies go back decades. Although they have not undermined uptake of ADHD at present—far from it—the "imperfect translations" have potential to pull support away from the current understanding and practice, opening the door to alternatives.

Co-Construction of ADHD: The Allies

Since the 1960s, an intricate network of allies has promoted a refined understanding of ADHD and ways to "manage" it. Although there have been prominent players in this process, there is no clear leader, and many constituencies have taken part.

Education, Special Education

Teachers require both attention and discipline (rule-following) from students. But some students do not pay attention in class or fail to follow instructions about staying in their seats, completing their assignments, waiting their turn, and so forth. These children present a twofold difficulty for their teachers: the children's own learning tends to lag behind that of their peers, and their activity level and distractibility disrupt the classroom. Both difficulties—especially the disruptive behaviors—tend to increase teacher stress (Greene, Beszterczey, Katzenstein, Park, & Goring, 2002). A school social worker, writing in the 1970s, when diagnosing and treating "hyperactivity" (a now-passé term for ADHD; see Chapter 1) was becoming more common, describes the situation:

> Teachers are trained to instruct students using skills that require the student to attend, function, and produce within a given structure and time limitations. Hyperactive children are problems for teachers who, in turn, are problems for hyperactive children because these children do not possess the abilities to learn successfully in the manner specified by the school... The interactional effects of the student with the teacher and the class result in a secondary series of problems affecting everyone (Renstrom, 1976, 97, 99).

The hyperkinetic child's behavior disrupted the classroom, threatening the teacher's professional and personal self-respect, and at least for some teachers it also threatened job security because ability to control the classroom was a prerequisite for a good teaching evaluation (Renstrom, 1976). Educators tested behavior modification strategies for hyperkinetic children grouped in nontraditional classrooms (Krauch, 1971; Miller, 1973) or remaining in traditional classrooms (Hackett, 1975), but these were difficult to implement and not widely successful.

To address these problems, a school–physician–parent alliance began to form in the 1960s. Parents brought children who were disruptive in school (or at home) to clinicians; physicians more commonly diagnosed "hyperkinesis" or "minimal brain dysfunction" (another ADHD precursor; see Chapter 1) and prescribed Ritalin (methylphenidate), which was approved by the U. S. Food and Drug Administration (FDA) in 1955. The 1980 revision of the DSM, DSM-III (American Psychiatric Association, 1980), cemented the alliance by codifying the concerns of teachers (and parents) about school behavior in the diagnostic criteria for the disorder, which was then called attention deficit disorder (ADD). No longer as vaguely defined, the diagnostic criteria now included such behaviors as "difficulty concentrating on schoolwork (American Psychiatric Association, 1980, 43)," "frequently calls out in class (44)," and "has difficulty staying seated (44)."

Meanwhile, the education system responded by initiating and gradually standardizing practices to address ADHD-associated academic and behavioral difficulties. Increasingly over the '70s, '80s, and '90s, teachers became intimately involved in detecting and managing ADHD-associated behaviors. Teachers or other school personnel suggested ADHD testing to a child's parent(s) or guardian(s) based on observations of classroom behavior and/or struggles with academic work; and in the DSM-III, priority is given to teacher reports of children's difficulties over those of parents, because of teachers' "greater familiarity with age-appropriate norms (American Psychiatric Association, 1980, 43)." As diagnoses increased, the U.S. Department of Education aimed to identify practices that would accord with education's key goals and core institutional values, and that could be integrated inexpensively into the existing school structure (Carlson, Hales, Burcham, & Challman, 1993). The goal was to identify "parents, health care professionals, school personnel, researchers, and clinicians" as "stakeholders" (allies?), who should be included in shaping the educational system's responses to ADD/ADHD-diagnosable individuals. Today, classroom teachers often suggest assessment, and they frequently complete a checklist of behaviors that the evaluating clinician incorporates into his/her assessment. The much higher diagnosis rates among younger children in classrooms (Elder, 2010; Evans, Morrill, & Parente, 2010) likely reflects the continuing influence of educators' needs on diagnostic practice.

After students have been diagnosed, teachers are often closely integrated into management strategies. If a child's behavior and learning problems are not severe, teachers (and parents—see below for more on their role as allies) may be satisfied with informal strategies, with or without medication use. Many ADHD-diagnosable children, however, require additional educational assistance. The next level of intervention for children whose learning difficulties can be tied to their ADHD status is development of an "accommodation plan," including an "individualized educational program" (IEP), in compliance with Section 504.[5] Typically carried out in a general classroom, accommodations may include simple interventions such as having the child's desk close to the teacher's. More teacher-intensive techniques include ADHD-appropriate conduct of lessons (for example, including quick feedback or additional explanations), or completing "Daily Report Cards" that communicate the child's behavior to the parent(s)/guardian(s). Extra use of peer co-tutoring is another option, giving the ADHD-diagnosed child opportunities for skill practice and interaction with others (U.S. Department of Education, 2006).

More severely symptomatic children qualify for special education services if they meet criteria outlined in the Individuals with Disabilities Education Act of 2004 (IDEA, 2004). Special education categories do not correspond directly to DSM categories, but ADHD-diagnosed children may qualify under one or more categories, depending on comorbidities.[6] An ADHD-diagnosed child who also has learning disabilities may qualify for services under the "specific learning disability" category; those who have comorbid conduct disorder or oppositional defiant disorder may qualify under the "emotional disturbance" category. The most common and straightforward classification, though, is the "other health impairment" (OHI) category.[7] In two key translations of education practice to psychiatric and scientific concepts, OHI was interpreted to include ADD/ADHD beginning in 1991 (Aleman, 1991; Wright, 1995) and the language of IDEA '97 added ADD/ADHD.[8]

Unlike Section 504 designation, special education classification brings additional federal funding to the schools.[9] The students' expenses are also higher than those of non-disabled children, which, on average, totaled $6,566 per child in 1999–2000 (Chambers, Shkolnik, & Perez, 2003). The OHI category is probably a good proxy for expenses for educating children with relatively severe ADHD symptoms in public school settings, because a high percentage of OHI-classified children are ADHD-diagnosed.[10] If this is so, then, educational expenses for these ADHD-diagnosed children—that is, for (very roughly) 10% of those who are diagnosed[11]—is $13,229 (Chambers et al., 2003)—more than twice that of their non-diagnosable peers. This level of spending is controversial, as is the sharp increase in the number of students so categorized since 1991, the year IDEA was interpreted to include ADD/ADHD. Nationally, growth in that category from 1992 to 2002 was 319% President's Commission on Special Education, 2002), concomitant with the growth in ADHD diagnosis and drug treatment in that period (the increase in diagnostic rates between 1990 and 2000 was approximately 400% to 500%, and stimulant prescriptions increased by about 800% in the same period [Mayes & Bokhari, 2002; Robison, Sclar, Skaer, & Galin, 1999].)

Thus, educators have had a number of incentives for making ADHD a standard part of their practice. Dealing with burgeoning requests for Section 504 and IDEA accommodations is one. More centrally, though, solving the dual problems of below-par academic achievement and poor classroom control problems tied—and still ties—to core values of the institution. The idea that each child needs to be taught, whatever his or her difficulties, rests on promoting the present and future good of education for each child. In turn, this vision is based at least in part on another core value—that of equity. As one government report on special education puts it, "[S]pecial education has become one of the most important symbols of American compassion, inclusion and educational opportunity (President's Commission on Special Education, 2002)." Whatever behavioral or educational benefits stem from diagnosis and appropriate accommodation reinforce the uptake of ADHD, simultaneously strengthening the association of ADHD diagnosis with learning and behavior difficulties. In Latourian terms, at the same time as clinicians' and scientists' diagnostic criteria were translated to reflect educators' concerns, the educators' concerns were translated to reflect clinical and scientific language and practice.

Parents[12]

Parents are important allies of other stakeholders in the uptake and co-construction of the ADHD category. Many parents of ADHD-diagnosable children strongly desire to help their children who struggle with academics, classroom or social expectations for behavior, or social or family relationships—but the difficulties of helping may also cause frustration. Like those of the educators, the goals, expectations, and needs of parents co-construct the ADHD diagnostic criteria. For example, home-based problems such as "failure to follow through on parental requests and instructions (American Psychiatric Association, 1980, 41)" were included as symptoms in the DSM-III diagnostic criteria and in the descriptive preface to those criteria; current diagnostic criteria include similar behaviors.

Many parents actively voice their concerns and seek help from a teacher or from a physician. By doing so, the parents recruit teachers and/or physicians as allies. Often, parents seek a physician's help with the ADHD diagnosis in mind (Sax & Kautz, 2003).[13] Parents are also in charge of dispensing medicine, keeping track of side effects and efficacy, and monitoring a child's progress at home and at school, in coordination with the child's teacher.

But parents must also adapt their language and practice to that of the clinicians and scientists. Even at the diagnostic stage, the parent must fill out forms that translate their understanding and observations of their child into clinical language. For example, from a questionnaire concerning 6- to 12-year-olds at risk of ADHD, the parent needs to answer the question, does the child "never/sometimes/often/always have difficulty playing or engaging in leisure activities quietly?" To do this, the parent needs to consider his/her child's many activities and think: Does the child have *difficulty*? or Is s/he just not quiet? What is a "leisure activity" for my child? Quietly? *How* quietly? This and the many other questions on such forms structure observations of the child in a specific way.

After diagnosis and agreeing to treatment, parenting takes on practices—clinician visits, medicating, parent–teacher conferences, behavior modification techniques—that adapt family function to the ADHD category and its medical management. When many parents adapt in this way, the structures and procedures associated with the ADHD diagnosis are reinforced, as is the diagnostic category itself. This is another aspect of parents' role in co-constructing ADHD. When the treatment proves beneficial, the alliance—and DSM-defined ADHD—is further strengthened.

ADHD-Diagnosed Children and Adults

Until the late 1990s, ADHD was primarily a disorder of children. Because diagnosis and treatment decisions were made by parents and other adults, rather than by the child, the children were not themselves allies in promoting and solidifying ADHD.[14] In Latourian terms, they were more akin to actants, as it was their behavior being observed and interpreted according to specific tests, criteria, and manipulations in the clinic and schools. Even for adolescents in this era, the pressure of structures and expectations put in place by others complicates interpretation of their choices. The complex issues involved will be discussed more fully in Chapter 5.

More recently, however, the dynamic has begun to change. As of 2005, 1.7 million of the 5 million taking prescription medication for ADHD were adults (Anonymous, 2006a). And, while the rate of increase among children was sharp, but slowing (the number of prescriptions rose 46% between 2002 and 2010 (Zoler, 2010), a relative leveling after the 400% to 500% increase in the 1990s), among adults the increase was steeper, and there was no drop-off: in the 2000–2005 time period, prescriptions for those aged 20 to 44 years increased 139% (Anonymous, 2006a).

Although pressures analogous to those on children and teens drive some of the decisions, the recent uptake among adults also suggests an increased acceptability of the diagnosis among diagnosable individuals. Many ADHD-diagnosable individuals find that diagnosis and treatment help them cope with requirements of work, school, home, and relationships. Like the parents of ADHD-diagnosable children, adults translate their struggles to the clinical and scientific language of impairments, deficits, and malfunctions. Conversely, in a move reminiscent of the earlier codification of teachers' and parents' concerns as symptoms, the DSM-5 adds individuals' subjective symptoms of distraction by "unrelated thoughts" and being "uncomfortable being still for extended time" to the diagnostic criteria (American Psychiatric Association, 2013, 59-60; *see* Chapter 6 for more detail). A strengthened alliance may be the result.

Physicians[15]

In the 1970s, physicians faced a problem. Wanting help, frustrated parents brought their hard-to-manage children to doctor's offices, concerned about their limited success in school and with friends. Once a few studies showed that stimulant drugs sometimes improved behavior, doctors had a way to translate parents' concerns into clinical solutions, and they began to do so. Many physicians at the time remained skeptical of the nascent diagnostic category. Questions included the possibility of accurate diagnosis (Kenny et al., 1971): Could children with inextricably intertwined scholastic and behavioral disorders—but without classical signs of neurological disease—be distinguished from their normal peers (Wikler, Dixon, & Parker, 1970)? Some suggested that treatment in this setting could not be rational (Freeman, 1976) or safe (Charles & Froh, 1971; O'Donnell, 1971; Rapp, 1971; Schwartz et al., 1971; Willey, 1971). But others strongly supported recognition of the diagnosis, arguing that the syndrome was indeed "common," "real," and "significant" (Eisenberg, 1972)." Psychiatrist Leon Eisenberg concluded that treatment with stimulants was often mandatory, for the reason that "...our failure to understand cause and mechanism does not diminish the reality of the clinical phenomena and the personal suffering that confront us (Eisenberg, 1972, 710)."

The latter view won out, of course. Today, caring for ADHD-diagnosable individuals is part of daily practice for many physicians—especially those who care for children and adolescents, but increasingly for those caring for adults as well (Robison, Sclar, & Skaer, 2005). For many physicians, overarching values of compassion and support for individuals guide patient care, in which case treatment goals align with parents' or diagnosed individuals' perspectives (as opposed to those of educators, employers, etc.). Treatment may address an affected person's self-esteem, friendships, and sense of accomplishment, as well as goals such as meeting classroom and workplace expectations. The overarching medical values have been codified in the co-constructed ADHD in the term "impairment," which appears in the DSM's definition of mental disorder as well as in the ADHD diagnostic criteria specifically (see Chapter 1). The underlying ethical concerns reinforce the legitimacy and uptake of the diagnostic category in ways clinical science alone does not.

Focus on the individual patient also fosters an alliance among physicians, diagnosable individuals, parents, and teachers (because teachers are integrally involved in diagnosis and monitoring of treatment efficacy). Psychologists (see endnote 15) who provide additional forms of therapy may be allies as well; cross-referrals for multimodal care contribute to the network. Physicians and psychologists also rely on, and are thus allied with, researchers in various fields who provide updated or innovative information concerning etiology and treatment efficacy.

The economics of medical management also builds alliances. Even in the 1970s, "... as funds were made available and the 'epidemic' of cases and causes became more impressive, almost every conceivable field tried to participate in the bonanza" (Freeman, 1976, 14). Fields proposing etiologies relevant to their specialties included allergic medicine, ophthalmology, toxicology, genetics, and more. In Latourian terms, the specialists cultivated a role in the growing alliance, adapting their research and treatment goals to the perceived need (and therefore paying patients) and available research funding.

Complex economic influences continue. ADHD treatment is both a potential income source for clinicians and a target for increasing efficiency and cost-effectiveness of care. The cost of ADHD care is significant. One group estimates that the annual "cost of illness" for an ADHD-diagnosed adolescent, including health care, education, parents' lost work, and juvenile justice involvement, averages $14,576 each, of which $2,636 is health care and mental health care (Pelham, Foster, & Robb, 2007). An initial diagnostic work-up alone averages $2,000 (Diller, 2006), and ongoing care and adjustments in treatment are needed: As we saw in Chapter 1, more than 3 million office visits concerning ADHD take place annually for those under 18 (National Center for Health Statistics, 2006; c.f. endnote 3, Chapter 1), and the 1.7 million adults prescribed ADHD medications also must receive care. Insurance coverage defrays some costs for insured individuals and families and compensates treating clinicians. It helps establish a predictable economic exchange, laying the groundwork for economic incentives that stabilize the treatment category and the alliances.

The authors of the Multimodal Treatment of ADHD trial (MTA) argue that "medical management" is, for most ADHD-diagnosed children, the most cost-effective of the representative treatments they assessed (Jensen et al., 2005).[16] The Multimodal Treatment of ADHD trial (MTA) is a large, ongoing, federally funded study comparing "medical management," in which drug dosages were carefully titrated during follow-up visits; intensive behavioral treatment without drugs; combined medical management and behavioral treatment; and "community care," in which ADHD-diagnosed children were referred to community physicians for treatment—in practice, this meant that the children tended to receive prescriptions, but not intensive behavioral therapy or sophisticated drug titration. Costs per child for the 14-month period of the initial trial were, respectively, $1,180, $6,988, $7,327, and $1,071, respectively. Factors such as parents' preference for the behavioral management treatment option complicate alliance formation. Yet, because "medical management" is in sync with DSM-defined ADHD, the coextension of clinical and economic efficiency suggests a further reason that ADHD (and the physician's role in the alliance) have been stabilized.

Notably, the economic alliance includes the pharmaceutical industry (see below for more about their role) and tends to exclude psychologists (see endnote 15). Physicians and the pharmaceutical industry are both integrally involved in providing relatively inexpensive drug therapy, while psychological care, although it arguably improves on medical care alone, adds greatly to costs. The MTA analysts do lukewarmly suggest that, "For some children with comorbid disorders, it may be relatively cost-effective to provide combination treatment (Jensen et al., 2005, 1635)." But this is hardly the warm endorsement they offer of "medical management" over "community care":

> ...in view of the greater costs incurred by ADHD children than healthy children for medical costs ($1,000–2,000 per year) and for auto accidents ($3,000) and their increased use of other expensive programs (special education services, juvenile justice, etc.), the modest incremental costs for more effective versus less effective programs (e.g., $360 for intensive medication management versus standard community care) seem easily justified and potentially a wise investment. (Jensen et al., 2005,1635)

In other words, clinical medicine, in concert with the drug companies, provides "more effective" treatment *and* can save money for parents, the auto and medical insurance industries, public education, and the juvenile justice system. This translates a medical success—improved SNAP ratings—to broad-scale social concerns.

The connections are yet more explicit in the public health arena, where ADHD draws attention through its association with a number of public health issues. ADHD-diagnosed people have higher risks of smoking, substance abuse, and severe injury (National Institutes of Health,1998; DiScala, Lescohier, Barthel, & Li, 1998; Rowland, Lesesne, & Abramowitz, 2002); high medical costs (the healthcare costs of ADHD-diagnosed children and adolescents, including but not limited to treatment for ADHD per se, are double those of nondiagnosable individuals; Leibson, Katusic, Barbaresi, Ransom, & O'Brien, 2001); and their family members also have excess healthcare costs (Birnbaum et al., 2005). Summarizing, the report of a 1998 NIH consensus conference states, "...these individuals consume a disproportionate share of resources and attention from the health care system, criminal justice system, schools, and other social service agencies...Moreover, ADHD, often in conjunction with coexisting conduct disorders, contributes to societal problems such as violent crime and teenage pregnancy" (National Institutes of Health, 1998, 9).

The translation of ADHD from the DSM-defined ADHD's "biological dysfunction in the individual" (*see* Chapter 1) to "public health problem," widens the scope, description, and types of problems associated with the disorder. In this new context, ADHD is called on to explain population-wide phenomena such as healthcare expenses ("conservatively estimated at $3.3 billion annually" for diagnosable individuals; Centers for Disease Control and Prevention, 2005, 847) and social ills from teen pregnancy to violent crime. Literature on the epidemiology of ADHD often first cites correlations between ADHD and various problems in society and then calls for more study *and* for more effective detection and treatment efforts (Biederman et al., 2006; National Institutes of Health, 1998; Kessler et al., 2006).

Drawing these connections—or, in Latour's framework, making these translations—in new contexts helps co-construct the predominant understanding of ADHD, incorporating into that understanding public health problems such as accidents, substance abuse, and violence. With ADHD as a common enemy, public health workers and researchers join clinicians and others in the network, all seeking to address overlapping problems in their realms of influence and concern. Once again, the (partially) shared goals have the intertwined results of contributing to the co-construction of ADHD and reinforcing and stabilizing the category and the practices concerning it.

Pharmaceutical Companies

Although many businesses profit from ADHD in various ways, such as selling tailored educational materials, it is safe to say that the extraordinary profits made by pharmaceutical companies from the increase in diagnosis of ADHD and its drug treatments have outstripped others' gains. To take one example, Shire Pharmaceuticals, based in the United Kingdom, has been highly dependent on Adderall and Adderall XR sales. The company's net sales in 2003, for example, were $1.2 billion—$536 million of that from the Adderall franchise (Breitstein, 2004). Its profits that year were $283 million, or 19.7% (Berberich, 2006).

Revenues like this make the pharmaceutical industry an eager ally and recruiter. (Individuals within the industry might of course have other motivations.) The drug companies pursue multiple means to increase awareness and sales of their products. For example, efforts to translate problems into the language of ADHD (and other mental illnesses) have been quite consciously undertaken by drug companies. As Elliott (2003) puts it, "...the key to selling psychiatric drugs is to sell the illnesses they treat" (123). In successfully selling the illness, pharmaceutical companies enroll parents, diagnosable individuals, clinicians, the insurance industry, government officials, and scientists as allies—and as profit producers. In the case of ADHD and its nosological precursors, such practices have been established at least since the 1970s. In 1971, a series of letters to *The New England Journal of Medicine* had expressed concern that drug company manipulation of physicians in the interest of profit were driving the rapid increase in stimulant prescriptions (most ADHD medications are stimulants). Howard Cohn of Ciba Pharmaceutical Company, then manufacturer of Ritalin, responded in the *Journal*, "Ciba has not 'embarked on an extremely expensive and skillfully designed advertising campaign': rather, we spend considerable time and effort in alerting practicing physicians to the existence of [ADHD precursor] minimal brain dysfunction as an entity, emphasizing the complex and often obscure symptomatology of the disease (Cohn, 1971, 1150)." This "time and effort" by the drug companies forges alliances between the drug company and the physicians, but also, secondarily, with ADHD-diagnosable individuals and their caregivers who use or purchase the drugs.

Today's version of this practice is to sell the disease directly to patients and their caregivers in addition to "alerting" physicians. Slogans such as Strattera's "from frustration to focus," or Adderall's "building an adult ADHD success story" are promoted via various media. In these advertisements, pharmaceutical companies position ADHD as an explanation for people's problems, and medication as the solution to struggles toward educational, vocational, and social success. Although the ads are directed at diagnosable individuals, caregivers, or clinicians, they speak, too, to educators, employers, and the wider society, promising an easy answer to problems of schools, the workplace, and the street. In these efforts, pharmaceutical companies also tangentially address officials in charge of funding for scientific and medical research, familiarizing them with the importance of ADHD as a medical and social problem. In addition, pharmaceutical companies spend enormous amounts of money on drug research (unfortunately, the exact figures are elusive [Angell, 2004]), thus creating research opportunities in the ADHD field, as well as guiding the type (and to some extent the results) of research that is done.[17] Further, they fund advocacy groups such as Children and Adults with Attention-Deficit/Hyperactivity Disorder (CHADD) and National Alliance on Mental Illness (NAMI) that support and lobby for those who have mental illnesses. In this way, the drug companies support and recruit allies who lobby for social recognition—especially destigmatization[18]—of specific mental disorders, along with access to drug and other treatments. In crafting their messages and directing their support in specific directions, drug companies contribute substantially to the co-construction and stabilization of DSM-defined ADHD, as well as directly promoting the uptake and institutionalization of drug treatment.

Advocacy Groups

Several groups support and lobby on behalf of ADHD-diagnosed individuals. The largest is CHADD, which was formed in 1987 as a support group for parents with ADHD-diagnosable children. The organization's stated aims are to provide support, education, and advocacy on behalf of those who have ADHD. It has about 20,000 members, 2,000 of whom are professionals who provide clinical services to those who have ADHD.[19]

CHADD's communications and activities link and/or draw support from a number of ADHD stakeholders. For example, CHADD conveys information from scientists and clinicians to its "lay" members and the broader public. One such forum is an "education initiative" called "ASK: AD/HD. Science. Knowledge," which is "designed to educate policymakers, the media, and the American public about the science behind AD/HD." A goal of this effort is to reduce stigma concerning ADHD, which CHADD sees as a deterrent to seeking assistance for the disorder.[20] The organization also cites connections with government, exemplified by its National Resource Center on AD/HD, which is funded by the Centers for Disease Control (CDC). It is tied to clinical medicine and psychology via its professional members, national meeting, education efforts, and "cooperative working agreements" with the American Academy of Child and Adolescent Psychiatry and the American Academy of Pediatrics.

In Latourian terms, these efforts are of course intended to recruit allies. But it is not entirely clear which constituency is the driving force behind CHADD's efforts. To the extent that CHADD remains a "grassroots" organization, adult ADHD-diagnosed individuals and parents of ADHD-diagnosed children are effecting CHADD's alliances. However, CHADD is funded to a significant degree by the pharmaceutical industry: According to its 2008–2009 income and expenditure report,[21] 26.6% ($1,174,626) of its annual budget consisted of pharmaceutical company support. The professional membership may also be influential.

CHADD helps stabilize DSM-defined ADHD by its activities on behalf of those diagnosed, and by its support of government, education, and healthcare policies that incorporate the category. But it is important that CHADD also requires that understanding of ADHD be both *destigmatized* and *supportive*. This nuance is important and is a contribution by CHADD, among others, to the co-construction of present views of ADHD. However, destigmatization and support do not necessarily track together, as we will see in the second section of this chapter and again in Chapter 5.

Science

In explaining science's contributions to the predominant understanding of ADHD, Chapter 2 discussed science as if it were largely independent of social influence. In fact, however, science and scientists are as much in need of allies as people in other social groups. One reason science needs allies is that it needs funding. Research funding promotes growth in knowledge of a topic and continuity of the research program, and it enables success of individual scientists. Funding of research that has practical applications is a crucial give-and-take between science and society: Scientists need the funding, and social pressure exists to solve a problem. Scientists, through grant writing, try to convince funding agencies that their approach will contribute to a solution. If the funding agency is convinced, it grants an award. In the United States, some of the funds used to study ADHD come from government sources. A simple search of the NIH's Computer Retrieval of Information on Scientific Projects

(CRISP) site (http://crisp.cit.nih.gov) by year, using the phrase "attention deficit hyperactivity disorder" and looking only at the category "Research Grants" reveals that the NIH awarded an average of 105 federal grants annually for study of ADHD in the years 2000 through 2006; the peak year was 2005, with 144 grants awarded. The dollar figure on these awards held relatively constant over the same period, at an average of $107 million annually. Private funding, particularly by pharmaceutical companies, likely outstrips the NIH figure significantly (Angell, 2004).[22]

Science needs the world's cooperation in other ways, too. Philosopher Joseph Rouse explains that to achieve scientific success, scientists and their "applied" colleagues need both a laboratory and a changed world (Rouse, 1987). For example, scientists developed vaccines in controlled experiments conducted in laboratory "microworlds (ix)," but demonstration of real-world effectiveness[23] comes only after practices of physician education, accessible clinics, and immunization laws have been established. Clearly, scientists do not develop these systems on their own. The actions of millions of parents, clinicians, educators, and so forth, who support or undertake vaccination drive the social changes that prevent disease. Equally clearly, effective social changes also depend on careful laboratory investigations. In this way, changes in the social landscape and in the science are interdependent: "Neither the world nor our ways of being in it come 'first.' Each becomes determinate only in relation to the other (157)."

For the sciences of ADHD, the give-and-take began in earnest in the mid-twentieth century, as scientists recognized that the needs of parents, educators, and clinicians provided an opportunity. They responded by studying causation and treatment of minimal brain dysfunction, hyperkinesis, and finally ADHD and ADD, convincing educators and clinicians to be their allies. Researchers recommended and promoted practices they believed would potentiate the effective application of ADHD theory: proper drug dosages, efficient referral and identification mechanisms in schools, accurate techniques of clinical assessment, and so forth. Each of these came to allow a degree of consistency in determining who is ADHD-diagnosable, choosing which individuals receive medication or other interventions (and which form, for how long, etc.), administering the interventions, and tracking whether the interventions succeed according to established criteria. Other practices have been built on this groundwork, including criteria for physician, teacher, and parent education, and reimbursement to clinicians for treatment. Once a practice is adopted, scientists often continue to study it, helping to find ways to improve it.

But notice the order in which the steps take place: the initial laboratory efficacy, then the changes in practice, *then* the demonstration of (real world) effectiveness. Granted, the changes can be incremental; still, the non-scientist allies need to take a "leap of faith." Latour suggests that the French hygienists believed Pasteur without question, with "trust so great it must have been based on something else" (Latour, 1988, 26). For the educators, clinicians, parents, and others who allow themselves to be recruited by (and to recruit) scientists, that "something else" is the hope for a solution to their problems. Entering the alliance, though, requires accepting the cumulative definition of ADHD. People are willing to do this in part because of the pre-existing imprimatur of science: scientific approaches are importantly successful in many arenas, and the promise exists for ADHD as well. In the process, the needs of scientists, as well as educators and clinicians, contribute to the co-construction of ADHD.

Section Conclusion

Each constituency has reasons to accept DSM-defined ADHD, to work that category into its own practices, and to ally with others who find the category useful. In each case, uptake is based on core needs or other values of the institution, group, or individual. As we have seen, each group also translates its concerns into those of one or more other groups, forging a network of alliances among and between each of the constituencies. In the process, the understanding of ADHD shifts, as do institutional and social structures—that is, society shifts the understanding of ADHD *and* the understanding of ADHD changes society. Each constituency takes initiatives in this regard, so that no group can be considered "the" driving force behind ADHD. Rather, the groups jointly take up and stabilize the category and associated practices. Jointly, the influence has been powerful, as uptake of the diagnosis suggests. In Latourian terms, ADHD has a long and strong network.

Controversies and Unsolved Problems: Destabilizers and Adversaries

DSM-defined ADHD serves many needs and interests, both creating and stabilizing the category. An objection to this interpretation is lurking, however. The focus on alliances seems to downplay the multiple controversies that have beset ADHD for decades—changes in scientific theories, manipulation by drug companies, concerns about overdiagnosis, labeling, medicalization, and more. These influences, too, are significant, and it may be that, over time, the alliance that has been built up around ADHD will fail. This section discusses some of the countervailing considerations that could erode DSM-defined ADHD's stability and/or the alliances built around the concept.

Imperfect Translation

One general factor that can tend to eat away at alliances is partial mismatch among the needs and goals of various constituencies. When, for example, special education goals and criteria do not neatly align with clinical diagnoses, parents' hopes for their children don't coincide with the availability of a marketable drug, or individuals' goals and values depart from public health priorities, the failures of translation may diminish the rationale for alliances.

One prominent goal for parents, teachers, and ADHD-diagnosable individuals is improved academic achievement. Large numbers have found the help they needed through diagnosis and various interventions. Yet one of the important gaps between expectations and demonstrated effectiveness is that no specific intervention—educational, behavioral, or pharmacological—has yet been shown to improve academic achievement of ADHD-diagnosed individuals over the long term (National Institutes of Health, 1998; Jensen et al., 2007; MTA Cooperative Group, 2004; Purdie, Hattie, & Carroll, 2002; Xu, Reid, & Steckelberg, 2002). At present, concerns about this *possible* lack of effectiveness are based largely on absence of evidence rather than negative studies, because few long-term studies have been completed. Even the MTA, which *is* a long-term study that includes academic endpoints, only includes data from specific protocols and measures. This means that although the 3-year follow-up shows *no* differences among treatment groups on any measure, including reading scores and social skills; *all* treatment groups showed improvement over baseline; and there is no non-treatment group for comparison; the authors caution that, "It would be incorrect to conclude from these results that treatment makes no difference or is not worth pursuing" (Jensen et al., 2007, 1000). Still, the lack of evidence for long-term academic improvement means that central problems for parents and educators have not yet been resolved by interventions based on DSM-defined ADHD.

Diagnosis and treatment can disrupt other parental goals and perspectives as well, as Singh's structured interviews with parents of ADHD-diagnosed boys attest (Singh, 2005). Singh notes deep conflicts between parents' concepts of masculinity, self-actualization, success, authenticity, and personal freedom and their concepts of diagnosis and pharmacological treatment.

The parents Singh interviewed did have their children under medical treatment, but many parents opt out of this choice. It is not much of a leap to suggest that when conflicts such as those observed by Singh are deep enough, the medical solution is unattractive relative to the parents' values or goals. The concerns of this minority (in the United States) of parents are discussed further in Chapter 5.

ADHD-diagnosable individuals may have reservations similar to those of the parents just described, in which case they not necessarily allies of medicine. If it is correct that 17.5 million people are diagnosable,[24] there may be a significant number who choose not to embrace the diagnosis.[25] The views of members of the consumer/survivor/ex-patient (c/s/x) movement, although they typically have mental disorders more debilitating than ADHD, provide insight into individual reasons to reject psychiatric categories or practices (Morrison, 2005). Some c/s/x'ers reject psychiatry entirely; others think treatment benefits them but object to specific psychiatric practices. In the latter case, the individuals resist "...the imposition of definitions and constraints on their lives, even if they agree['d' omitted] with the definitions themselves" (Morrison, 2005, 54). The goal is a libertory rejection of the stigma of psychiatric illness, which c/s/x'ers see as deriving from the labeling by professionals and from social attitudes toward the diagnoses and people who have them. Three routes to rejecting the stigma are "reject[ing] the stigma inherent in the illness"—that is, to embrace the illness as a legitimate way of being; "reject[ing] the illness itself"—denying that specific traits and behaviors constitute an illness; and "reject[ing] the notion that the illness is 'who they are'" (Morrison, 2005, 12). Denying the authority of professionals to "define" them is one approach to such liberation; the more radical reject the definitions or psychiatry's efforts to control individuals.

Similar issues are raised with respect to ADHD. Concerns with "labeling" are common (Burns, 2000; Eide & Eide, 2006; Parens & Johnston, 2009). In addition, the role of DSM-defined ADHD in establishing a framework and means for changing an individual's behavior arguably makes medical control also control of the diagnosed individual—a control some resist (Conrad & Potter, 2000; Conrad & Schneider, 1992 [1980]). Long-standing discomfort with these issues—particularly as it concerns children who are not making diagnosis and treatment decisions for themselves—may lead either ADHD-diagnosable individuals or parents of diagnosable children to embrace a "different" way of being, despite manifest difficulties; to "reject the illness"; or to deny professional authority to control or define them or their children. By doing so, they clearly fall out of the ADHD alliance.

Advocacy groups like CHADD see themselves engaged in the destigmatizing project on behalf of ADHD-diagnosed individuals, as does the analogous patient advocacy group, the National Alliance on Mental Illness (NAMI). Yet c/s/x'ers see the NAMI form of advocacy—pushing, according to NAMI's website,[26] for "...the eradication of mental illnesses and to the improvement of the quality of life of all whose lives are affected by these diseases"—as maintaining the position of oppression. This nuanced concern questions the advocacy of what c/s/x'ers call "NAMI Mommies" on behalf of the mentally ill. These critics see the focus on "eradication" as an attempt to undermine the legitimacy of their way of being. Again, a parallel argument could be made against CHADD and other ADHD-advocacy groups. To the extent ADHD-diagnosable individuals or their caregivers agree with this argument, the alliance between them and the advocacy group is weakened.

The translation of the problems of parents, educators, clinicians, and the other allies to public health concerns is also imperfect; similarly, the reverse translation, of public health problems to sequelae of ADHD, is flawed. Interventions based on the ADHD paradigm can only provide partial answers to problems considered pressing from a public health perspective. For example, although "having" ADHD is associated with the public health issues of smoking, substance abuse, risky sexual behaviors, vehicle accidents, and youth violence, only *some* smokers, violent offenders, and others at risk have ADHD. Thus, interventions for ADHD can only solve part of the problem. Nor is there adequate data to specify preventive efforts, although a need for these has been voiced (Rowland et al., 2002). ADHD-prevention efforts might someday target risk factors identified in epidemiological work—currently, correlations of ADHD with maternal smoking, lead exposure, television viewing, video games, and pesticide consumption have been observed (Bouchard, Bellinger, Wright, & Weisskopf, 2010; Christakis, Zimmerman, DiGiuseppe, & McCarty, 2004; Linnet et al., 2005; Swing, Gentile, Anderson, & Walsh, 2010; Woodruff et al., 2004)—but data and systems are not yet in place to focus such efforts. It is also the case that although government initiatives have targeted ADHD identification and treatment, and research funding has been consistent over the past decade, the disorder is not a top priority, as it is for many allies. For example, the Public Health Service's "Healthy People 2010" and "Healthy People 2020" initiatives state a number of goals for mental health care, but none targets ADHD explicitly (U.S. Department of Health and Human Services, 2000; U.S. Department of Health and Human Services, 2010).

Some of the imperfect translations just described may also be expressed as concerns about medicalization, the idea that too much human behavior or distress is being categorized as disease. Chapter 1 covers details. Briefly, anti-medicalizers object to one or more hallmarks of the predominant model of ADHD, in which ADHD is a categorically defined, biological dysfunction in an individual. We have seen that this model tends to dichotomize ADHD-diagnosable people from "normal" people and to downplay social, relational, or educational solutions to ADHD-associated problems while emphasizing drug therapy. Thus, some anti-medicalizers object to dichotomization, some to attributions of "dysfunction," others to insufficient focus on sociopolitical perspectives, yet others to medication use; they may question the validity of the DSM-defined ADHD, of interventions based on it, or the clinical structures that address ADHD. The rationale for their concern varies, depending on the particular behavior or symptom being medicalized and depending on other values or goals of the critic. Critics may belong to any constituency from which allies are recruited (with the exception of advocacy groups and the pharmaceutical industry, composed of self-selected pro-medicalizers); their critical stance makes them non-allies, or even adversaries, of DSM-defined ADHD.

Pharmacotherapy, Pharmaceutical Companies

Many of the reasons people choose to reject or question pharmaceutical therapy are specific to particular drugs, based on the drug's ineffectiveness against symptoms or traits of concern, unwanted side effects, or long-term risks. Officers in drug enforcement and public health officials voice concerns about the potential for abuse or diversion of stimulant medications (Drug Enforcement Administration, 2005). Such criticisms do not involve criticism of the predominant ADHD paradigm more generally.

However, others offer criticisms that do raise concerns about present practice in the alliance. Critics argue that pharmaceutical company involvement biases medical research and care (Diller, 2005; Lemmens, 2004; Lexchin, Bero, Djulbegovic, & Clark, 2003; Melander, Ahlqvist-Rastad, Meijer, & Beermann, 2004; Peppercorn, Blood, Winer, & Partridge, 2007). The very high-profit pharmaceutical industry is closely involved in physician education and pharmaceutical research (Angell, 2004, 30).[27] The concern is that the drug companies' marketing, research, and lobbying efforts color physician attitudes and the information available to clinicians in a way that is good for pharmaceutical business but not necessarily good for people. In various constituencies, suspicion of the pharmaceutical industry's motives and tactics diminishes trust in drug companies as potential allies.

Equity

Another set of concerns is that current implementation of diagnosis, treatment, or other forms of management or accommodation is unfair, or at least questionably equitable on various grounds. Such arguments do not directly threaten an idealized version of DSM-defined ADHD. However, they do affect the alliance around the currently predominant understanding. The alliance has accepted a category known to have imprecise boundaries, multiple comorbidities, and no physical markers, and many concerns about equity are tied to these imprecisions and unknowns. If doubtful or negative consequences follow from adopting the current ADHD model, potential allies may be dissuaded from accepting it.

Within the school system, for example, solutions to ADHD-associated behavioral and academic difficulties have introduced long-standing conflicts among potential allies over the expense of implementation. According to a report to Congress in 1991, parents enthusiastically embraced the proposed expansion of IDEA to specifically include ADHD-diagnosable children, but school administrators did not. The National Education Association, the National Association of State Directors of Special Education, and the National School Boards Association also opposed the change. The concerns were that (1) children who needed assistance were already being served under traditional special education labels; (2) the diagnostic category was too controversial; and (3) including ADHD would overburden special education, directing resources away from those who needed them more (Aleman, 1991). Despite the administrators' opposition, IDEA was amended in 1997 to make ADHD-diagnosable children eligible. The sharp increase in numbers in special education's other health impairment (OHI) category since then has generated additional controversy. Advocates for ADHD diagnosis and for diagnosed individuals often view the increase positively, in that it indicates an attempt to address children's needs. Indeed, some advocates think that the increase is inadequate—for example, a position paper formulated by a coalition of mental-health-advocacy and other groups coordinated by CHADD concluded in 2003 that IDEA '97 was not being fully implemented or funded, thus leaving many eligible children without adequate educational assistance (Children's Behavior Alliance, 2003).[28] Others, however, find the expansion unwarranted for a number of reasons, including expense or misdirection of funds (President's Commission on Special Education, 2002) and troubling expansion of attributions of failure (Burns, 2000).[29] These conflicting goals and suggested solutions fray the alliance and potentially destabilize DSM-defined ADHD.

Testing

Apparent inequities in accommodations granted to ADHD-diagnosable individuals for standardized testing also raise concerns. With appropriate documentation, students with an ADHD diagnosis and verified disability secondary to the diagnosis can take standardized admissions tests—including the SAT, ACT, GRE, LSAT, and MCAT—with extra time, over several days, or in a separate room. Up until 2002, test boards "flagged" their scores, alerting score recipients that the test had been given under special conditions and, presumably, discouraging abuse of the system. Under legal pressure from disability rights activists, however, test boards dropped the flagging (except in the case of the MCAT and LSAT); simultaneously, they increased requirements for documentation of disability considerably (Abrams, 2005; Anonymous 2006b). In theory, students whose ADHD is controlled adequately for school participation and testing, by medication or otherwise, are *not* eligible for accommodations, while those who have significant residual disability are eligible. But it is controversial whether theory and practice are in sync. Some argue that warranted accommodations have been denied (Abrams, 2005; Duffy, 2006); others argue that accommodations are sometimes granted too liberally (Abrams, 2005).

For example, nationally, those who receive SAT testing accommodations receive somewhat lower scores than standard-test takers. In Washington, D.C., however, reporting is not amalgamated over a whole state and so can more clearly reveal disparities. There, Abrams' research showed that after flagging ended, scores on untimed tests increased markedly, but standard test scores were static, resulting in a combined score 200 points higher (out of the SAT's 1600) for accommodated test-takers (Abrams, 2005). In Abram's analysis, what happened was that some students were inappropriately *not* granted accommodation, while others were given an unfair advantage by unwarranted "accommodation." In his words, "By abolishing any stigma that might come with a flagged test, while tightening access to special accommodations, the College Board has given new opportunities to the strategic, while leaving behind the less savvy and less financially well-endowed (unpaginated)." In one sign that this might have been occurring even before flagging ended, Abrams cites California data that wealthy districts such as Beverly Hills and Newport Beach had higher-than-average numbers of accommodated test-takers, while *none* of the 1,439 SAT-takers from Los Angeles's inner-city schools were granted accommodations.

Another strategy is also employed by the "savvy": developmental pediatrician Lawrence Diller cites a case he says is not unusual—a young woman and her family wanted Diller to renew her Adderall prescription in time for her SAT tests, despite the fact that she had not taken the drug for 6 years, and then only for a few months (Diller, 2006).

Among those critical of these practices, some embrace the diagnosis but abhor abuse of the system; others think that the imprecise diagnosis and useful medications invite abuse. Either can readily agree that accommodations, when given, should be appropriate and fair. However, this example in which the ADHD category is sometimes subject to abuse can erode confidence in the category itself, as well as in the practices around it, particularly for those who are predisposed to find the category invalid.

Race/Ethnicity

As far as is currently known, ADHD has the same prevalence across populations: no race, ethnicity, or national prevalences have yet been detected when diagnostic criteria are applied uniformly. Yet some (not all) studies of the issues find that in the United States, ADHD diagnosis and treatment rates differ by race or ethnicity. Based on survey and clinical reappraisal, Breslau et al. (2006) reported that adult Hispanics and non-Hispanic blacks are 70% less likely to have an ADHD diagnosis than are non-Hispanic whites. Similar findings have been reported in children, in a study that controlled for birth weight (low birth weight is associated with increased incidence of ADHD), income, and insurance coverage (low levels of the latter two serve as barriers to diagnosis and treatment). Hispanic and African-American (non-Hispanic) children are, likewise, 68% and 60% less likely to be diagnosed, respectively (Pastor & Reuben, 2005). The diagnosed children were also about 40% less likely to receive medication for their ADHD after controlling for income, insurance, and presence of other health concerns. Similarly, Bussing's research in Florida suggests that among children who have been identified as being at high risk of ADHD, caregivers of white children are more than twice as likely as those of black children to seek out diagnosis; the white children are also twice as likely to receive treatment (Bussing, Zima, Gary, & Garvan, 2003).

Researchers also observe different rates of classification in special education. Among children receiving special education services, whites are overrepresented relative to other racial/ethnic groups in the other health impairment (OHI) category (risk ratio: 1.63), which, as discussed above, consists largely of students whose educational disability is attributed to ADHD. In the special education category of "emotional disturbance" (more mixed in terms of DSM diagnoses but likely to have a large number of ADHD-diagnosable students who have comorbid oppositional defiant disorder or conduct disorder) blacks are overrepresented (risk ratio: 2.25) (President's Commission on Special Education, 2002).[30]

In interpreting these statistics, the problematic "play" in the diagnostic criteria must be kept in mind, and pinpointing reasons for the differential rates among racial/ethnic subgroups is fraught with ambiguities. The first complication for many of the statistics that indicate racial/ethnic differences in prevalence or treatment rates is whether the differences among groups are medically justified or whether the observed differences relate to biases or preferences in practice. Because there is no physical sign of the disorder, and because the diagnostic criteria are imprecise, the answer cannot be given with any precision at this time (Rowland et al., 2002). Even if the differences are based on documentable (but yet to be documented) variation in ADHD prevalence or severity, however, further questions of causality arise: What are the roles of differential socialization on ADHD traits and comorbidities, and how influential are these roles relative to the influence of genes or other biological factors? What factor(s) better explain the higher ADHD diagnosis (Pastor & Reuben, 2005), drug treatment (Pastor & Reuben, 2005; Stevens, Harman, & Kelleher, 2005), and special education (President's Commission on Special Education, 2002) rates among whites—access? social pressures in white culture? white parents' culturally determined power or savvy (Abrams, 2005)? Are lower rates among blacks and Hispanics (Breslau et al., 2006) signs of disconnection with schools, mistrust of the education or health care system, less knowledge about the disorder (Bussing, Gary, Mills, & Garvan, 2003; Bussing, Zima et al., 2003), barriers to seeking professional services (Bussing, Zima et al., 2003), or bias on the part of referring educators or clinicians? Or is lower prevalence evidence of a protective effect of adversity (Breslau et al., 2006), or an alternative explanatory model for behavior difficulties in use by caregivers (Bussing, Gary et al., 2003; Bussing, Zima et al., 2003)?

I cannot attempt to analyze these issues more closely here. What is clear is that many of the questions relevant to differences in diagnostic rates among races/ethnicities invoke the concerns voiced by critics discussed in this chapter and in Chapters 1 and 2: questions of diagnostic ambiguity, varying interpretations of behaviors and traits, and clashes of cultures and values have all been raised in the context of such criticisms. The possibilities of stereotyping or prejudice, and of differences among races/ethnicities in access to social or medical support, add potential destabilizers to the ADHD alliance. As with the test-taking issues, the disparities may not be relevant to ideal understanding of and practice concerning ADHD, but they could tend to erode support nonetheless.

Gender

As with race/ethnicity issues, I cannot here pursue gender issues in ADHD to the extent they deserve. But differences in diagnostic rates and targeted symptoms by gender raise issues similar to those presented by the differences among races/ethnicities. Historically, there has been a marked gender gap in ADHD diagnosis, with approximately four to five times as many primary school boys as girls diagnosed, but with a decreasing differential in high school and beyond. Recently, that gap in diagnosis and treatment has been closing. One theory to explain this is that scientists and clinicians now increasingly recognize ADHD's different presentation in girls and women (Gaub & Carlson, 1997; Graetz, Sawyer, & Baghurst, 2005; Greene et al., 2001; Hinshaw, Carte, Fan, Jassy, & Owens, 2007; Levy, Hay, Bennett, & McStephen, 2005; Newcorn et al., 2001; Ohan & Johnston, 2005; Quinn, 2005; Zalecki & Hinshaw, 2004). According to this theory, boys more often have hyperactive and impulsive symptoms, girls more often have more pronounced inattentive symptoms with little hyperactivity, making their diagnosis ADHD, inattentive type. Concerning treatment, women are also "catching up" to men. In the 19 years and younger age range, twice as many boys as girls are still prescribed drugs. But this ratio is decreased from that in the 1990s (in 1995, the ratio was 4.6:1; Zito, 2000), and among girls ages 10 to 19 years, the number of prescriptions increased 90% in the years 2000 to 2005, an increase 45% greater than that in boys. Because these gaps are narrowing, it appears that more women, girls, and their supporters are joining the alliance, encouraged by development of a more complex, nuanced view of ADHD.

But detecting gender differences in ADHD presentation, prevalence, and treatment response, like detecting race/ethnicity differences, is problematic by reason of the play in the diagnostic categories, coupled with differences in socialization and expectations for behavior or achievement (Sonuga-Barke, Dalen, & Remington, 2003). For that reason, an alternative consequence of gender is that research on women and girls will contribute to new stereotypes, the "ADHD woman/girl" and the "ADD woman/girl" to complement the protoypical male diagnosee. Those concerned about essentializing and dichotomizing may not yet have raised much outcry about this. But concerns about stereotyping common for prototypical ADHD apply similarly to the gendered versions. Potential thus exists for eventual fragmentation of current uptake.

Section Conclusion

Versions of many of the controversies discussed in this section have been ongoing for more than 40 years. The tenacity of the disagreements suggests that although DSM-defined ADHD is currently predominant, there is also continuing instability in the acceptance of that model and the social and medical structures for managing ADHD. To date, however, the co-constructed, DSM model of ADHD remains predominant, and no viable alternative has yet been proposed.

Conclusion

A complex mix of constituencies—the allies—have contributed to the present understanding of ADHD and to the intertwined strategies for managing ADHD-associated problems. The resulting concept/practice is what Latour calls a "durable whole" composed of "many assembled elements" (Latour, 1987, 122). In the face of factual and ethical uncertainties and controversies, the durability arises from the mutuality of the invested needs, interests, and empirical demonstrations. Pragmatic and ethical values involving education, employment, profit, professional advancement, compassion, egalitarianism, social control, efficiency, cost-effectiveness, self-esteem, independence, responsibility, social welfare, and undoubtedly others blend in the current construct, mixing with medical and scientific facts about ADHD. By addressing these many needs and interests (and the values that reflect them), ADHD enjoys the support and contributions of multiple allies. And in failing to address them, or in addressing the "wrong" ones, ADHD loses allies and gains adversaries. It remains to be seen just how durable the whole is—whether it will indeed continue to resist "all trials to break it apart" (122).

The mutuality has two overarching effects that need careful attention. First is the effect of social influence on scientific thought. Chapter 4 argues that the blending of scientific facts and social values does not leave the scientific facts pristinely value free. Instead, science embeds the social values. The strength of the co-constructed category, and its incorporated facts and values, also has significant effects on ADHD-diagnosable individuals. These effects are the subject of Chapter 5.

REFERENCES

Abrams, S. J. (2005). Unflagged SATs. *Education Next*, *3*(Summer), 42–44.

Aleman, S. R. (1991). *Special Education for Children with Attention Deficit Disorder: Current Issues. CRS Report for Congress.* (No. CRS-91-862-EPW). Washington, D.C.: Library of Congress, Congressional Research Service.

American Psychiatric Association (1980). *Diagnostic and Statistical Manual of Mental Disorders, 3rd ed.* Washington, D.C.: American Psychiatric Association.

American Psychiatric Association (2013). *Diagnostic and Statistical Manual of Mental Disorders: DSM-5* (5th ed.). Washington, DC: American Psychiatric Association.

Angell, M. (2004). *The Truth About the Drug Companies: How They Deceive Us and What to Do About It.* New York: Random House.

Anonymous (2006a). New data show adults continue to outpace children in growth of ADHD medication use. *Medco Media Room,* (March 21). Retrieved January 10, 2007, from http://medco.mediaroom.com/index.php?s=43&item=111

Anonymous (2006b). Services for students with disabilities. Retrieved March 5, 2007, 2007, from http://www.collegeboard.com/ssd/prof/eligible.html

Bastiaansen, D., Koot, H. M., Ferdinand, R. F., & Verhulst, F. C. (2004). Quality of life in children with psychiatric disorders: Self-, parent, and clinician report. *Journal of the American Academy of Child and Adolescent Psychiatry, 43*(2), 221–230.

Berberich, S. (2006). Buyout ends 2-year saga as Rockville drug firm stays. *Gazette. net,* (January 20, 2006). Retrieved December 4, 2007, from http://www.gazette.net/stories/012006/businew181405_31904.shtml

Biederman, J., & Faraone, S. V. (2005). Attention-deficit hyperactivity disorder. *The Lancet, 366,* 237–248.

Biederman, J., Monuteaux, M. C., Mick, E., Spencer, T., Wilens, T. E., Silva, J. M., et al. (2006). Young adult outcome of attention deficit hyperactivity disorder: a controlled 10-year follow-up study. *Psychological Medicine, 36,* 167–179.

Birnbaum, H. G., Kessler, R. C., Lowe, S. W., Secnik, K., Greenberg, P. E., Leong, S. A., et al. (2005). Costs of attention-deficit hyperactivity disorder (ADHD) in the US: Excess costs of persons with ADHD and their family members in 2000. *Current Medical Research and Opinion, 21*(2), 195–206.

Bouchard, M. F., Bellinger, D. C., Wright, R. O., & Weisskopf, M. G. (2010). Attention-deficit/hyperactivity disorder and urinary metabolites of organophosphate pesticides. *Pediatrics, 125*(6), e1270–e1277.

Breitstein, J. (2004). Think small, grow big. *Pharmaceutical Executive, 24*(7), 52–62.

Breslau, J., Aguilar-Gaxiola, S., Kendler, K. S., Su, M., Williams, D., & Kessler, R. C. (2006). Specifying race-ethnic differences in risk for psychiatric disorder in a USA national sample. *Psychological Medicine, 36,* 57–68.

Burns, M. K. (2000). Examining special education labels through attribution theory: a potential source for learned helplessness. *Ethical Human Sciences and Services, 2*(2), 101–107.

Bussing, R., Gary, F. A., Mills, T. L., & Garvan, C. W. (2003). Parental explanatory models of ADHD: Gender and cultural variations. *Social Psychiatry and Psychiatric Epidemiology, 38,* 563–575.

Bussing, R., Zima, B. T., Gary, F. A., & Garvan, C. W. (2003). Barriers to detection, help-seeking, and service use for children with ADHD symptoms. *The Journal of Behavioral Health Services and Research, 30*(2), 176–189.

Carlson, L., Hales, R., Burcham, B., & Challman, S. (1993). *Federal Resource Center for Special Education. Final Report.* Lexington, KY: Federal Resource Center for Special Education.

Centers for Disease Control and Prevention (2005). Prevalence of diagnosis and medication treatment for attention-deficit/hyperactivity disorder—United States, 2003. *MMWR, 54*(34), 842–847.

Chambers, J. G., Shkolnik, J., & Perez, M. (2003). *Total Expenditures for Students with Disabilities, 1999–2000: Spending Variation by Disability, Report 5.* Washington, D.C.: American Institutes for Research for the United States Department of Education, Office of Special Education Programs. Retrieved April 20, 2013, from http://csef.air.org/publications/seep/national/final_seep_report_5.pdf

Charles, A. F., & Froh, R. B. (1971). Methlyphenidate problems (cont.) (second letter). *The New England Journal of Medicine, 285*(17), 970.

Children's Behavior Alliance (2003). *In the Best Interests of All: A Position Paper of the Children's Behavioral Alliance.* Landover, MD: Children and Adults with Attention Deficit/Hyperactivity Disorder.

Christakis, D. A., Zimmerman, F. J., DiGiuseppe, D. L., & McCarty, C. A. (2004). Early television exposure and subsequent attentional problems in children. *Pediatrics, 113*(4), 708–713.

Cohn, H. D. (1971). Methylphenidate and minimal brain dysfunction (letter). *The New England Journal of Medicine, 285*(20), 1150.

Conrad, P., & Potter, D. (2000). From hyperactive child to ADHD adults: observations on the expansion of medical categories. *Social Problems, 47*(4), 559–582.

Conrad, P., & Schneider, J. W. (1992 (1980)). *Deviance and Medicalization: From Badness to Sickness.* Philadelphia, PA: Temple University Press.

Diller, L. (2005). Bitter pill: Ritalin and the growing influence of Big Pharma. *Psychotherapy Networker, 29*(1), unpaginated.

Diller, L. H. (2006). *The Last Normal Child: Essays on the Intersection of Kids, Culture, and Psychiatric Drugs.* Westport, CT: Praeger Publishers.

DiScala, C., Lescohier, I., Barthel, M., & Li, G. (1998). Injuries to children with attention deficit hyperactivity disorder. *Pediatrics, 102*(6), 1415–1421.

Drug Enforcement Administration, U.S. Department of Justice (2005). Drugs of Abuse; Chapter 5: Stimulants. Retrieved May 8, 2008, from http://www.usdoj.gov/dea/pubs/abuse/5-stim.htm#Methylphenidate

Duffy, S. P. (2006). Test taker sues to gain more LSAT time. *The Legal Intelligencer,* (December 26). Retrieved December 5, 2007, from http://www.law.com/jsp/article.jsp?id=1166695603211

Eide, B. L., & Eide, F. F. (2006). The mislabeled child. *The New Atlantis, 12*(Spring), 46–59.

Eisenberg, L. (1972). Symposium: behavior modification by drugs. III. The clinical use of stimulant drugs in children. *Pediatrics, 49*(5), 709–715.

Elder, T. E. (2010). The importance of relative standards in ADHD diagnoses: evidence based on exact birth dates. *J Health Econ, 29*(5), 641–656.

Elliott, C. (2003). *Better Than Well: American Medicine Meets the American Dream.* New York: W. W. Norton & Company.

Evans, W. N., Morrill, M. S., & Parente, S. T. (2010). Measuring inappropriate medical diagnosis and treatment in survey data: The case of ADHD among school-age children. *J Health Econ, 29*(5), 657–673.
Freeman, R. D. (1976). Minimal brain dysfunction, hyperactivity, and learning disorders: epidemic or episode? *School Review, 85*(1), 5–29.
Gaub, M., & Carlson, C. L. (1997). Gender differences in ADHD: A meta-analysis and critical review. *Journal of the American Academy of Child & Adolescent Psychiatry, 36*(8), 1036–1045.
Graetz, B. W., Sawyer, M. G., & Baghurst, P. (2005). Gender differences among children with DSM-IV ADHD in Australia. *Journal of the American Academy of Child & Adolescent Psychiatry, 44*(2), 159–168.
Greene, R. W., Beszterczey, S. K., Katzenstein, T., Park, K., & Goring, J. (2002). Are students with ADHD more stressful to teach? Patterns of teacher stress in an elementary school sample. *Journal of Emotional and Behavioral Disorders, 10*(2), 79–89.
Greene, R. W., Biederman, J., Faraone, S. V., Monuteaux, M. C., Mick, E., DuPre, E. P., et al. (2001). Social impairment in girls with ADHD: patterns, gender comparisons, and correlates. *Journal of the American Academy of Child & Adolescent Psychiatry, 40*(6), 704–710.
Hackett, R. (1975). In praise of praise. *American Education, 11*, 11–15.
Hinshaw, S. P., Carte, E. T., Fan, C., Jassy, J. S., & Owens, E. B. (2007). Neuropsychological functioning of girls with attention-deficit/hyperactivity disorder followed prospectively into adolescence: evidence for continuing deficits? *Neuropsychology, 21*(2), 263–273.
Individuals with Disabilities Education Improvement Act of 2004 (IDEA 2004), Pub. L. No. 108-446, 118 Stat. 2647 (2004).
Jensen, P. S., Arnold, L. E., Swanson, J. M., Vitiello, B., Abikoff, H. B., Greenhill, L. L., et al. (2007). 3-year follow-up of the NIMH MTA study. *Journal of the American Academy of Child and Adolescent Psychiatry, 46*(8), 989–1002.
Jensen, P. S., Garcia, J. A., Glied, S., Crowe, M., Foster, M., Schlander, M., et al. (2005). Cost-effectiveness of ADHD treatments: Findings from the Multimodal Treatment Study of Children with ADHD. *American Journal of Psychiatry, 162*(9), 1628–1636.
Kenny, T. J., Clemmens, R. L., Hudson, B. W., Lentz, G. A., Cicci, R., Nair, P. (1971). Characteristics of children referred because of hyperactivity. *The Journal of Pediatrics, 79*(4), 618–622.
Kessler, R. C., Adler, L., Barkley, R., Biederman, J., Conners, C. K., Demler, O., et al. (2006). The prevalence and correlates of adult ADHD in the United States: Results from the National Comorbidity Survey replication. *American Journal of Psychiatry, 163*(4), 716–723.
Krauch, V. (1971). Hyperactive engineering. *American Education, 7*, 12–16.
Latour, B. (1987). *Science in Action.* Cambridge, MA: Harvard University Press.
Latour, B. (1988). *The Pasteurization of France* (A. L. Sheridan, J, Trans.). Cambridge, MA: Harvard University Press.

Leibson, C. L., Katusic, S. K., Barbaresi, W. J., Ransom, J., & O'Brien, P. C. (2001). Use and costs of medical care for children and adolescents with and without attention-deficit/hyperactivity disorder. *JAMA, 285*(1), 60–66.

Lemmens, T. (2004). Leopards in the Temple: Restoring Scientific Integrity to the Commercialized Research Scene. *Journal of Law, Medicine, and Ethics, 32*(4), 641–657.

Leslie, L. K., & Wolraich, M. L. (2007). ADHD service use patterns in youth. *Ambul Pediatr, 7*(1 Suppl), 107–120.

Levy, F., Hay, D. A., Bennett, K. S., & McStephen, M. (2005). Gender Differences in ADHD Subtype Comorbidity. [References]. *Journal of the American Academy of Child & Adolescent Psychiatry, 44*(4), 368–376.

Lexchin, J., Bero, L. A., Djulbegovic, B., & Clark, O. (2003). Pharmaceutical industry sponsorship and research outcome and quality: systematic review. *British Medical Journal, 326,* 1167–1170.

Linnet, K. M., Wisborg, K., Obel, C., Secher, N. J., Thomsen, P. H., Agerbo, E., et al. (2005). Smoking during pregnancy and the risk for hyperkinetic disorder in offspring. *Pediatrics, 116*(2), 462–466.

Mayes, R., & Bokhari, F. (2002). *Rise of ADHD prevalence and psychostimulant use: a historical perspective.* Paper presented at the 130th Annual Meeting of APHA. Abstract retrieved April 20, 2013, from http://apha.confex.com/apha/130am/techprogram/paper_46109.htm

Melander, H., Ahlqvist-Rastad, J., Meijer, G., & Beermann, B. (2004). Evidence b(i)ased medicine—selective reporting from studies sponsored by pharmaceutical industry: review of studies in new drug applications. *British Medical Journal, 326,* 1171–1173.

Miller, F. (1973). Getting Billy into the game. *American Education, 9,* 22–27.

Morrison, L. J. (2005). *Talking Back to Psychiatry: The Psychiatric Consumer/Survivor/Ex-Patient Movement.* New York: Routledge.

MTA Cooperative Group (2004). National Institute of Mental Health multimodal treatment study of ADHD follow-up: 24-month outcomes of treatment strategies for attention-deficit/hyperactivity disorder. *Pediatrics, 113*(4), 754–761.

National Center for Health Statistics. (2006). *Health, United States, 2006, with Chartbook on Trends in the Health of Americans.* Hyattsville, MD: U.S. Government Printing Office.

National Institutes of Health (1998): *Diagnosis and treatment of attention deficit hyperactivity disorder (ADHD): NIH Consensus Statement.* Bethesda, MD: National Institutes of Health.

Newcorn, J. H., Halperin, J. M., Jensen, P. S., Abikoff, H. B., Arnold, L. E., Cantwell, D. P., et al. (2001). Symptom profiles in children with ADHD: effects of comorbidity and gender. *Journal of the American Academy of Child and Adolescent Psychiatry, 40*(2), 137–146.

O'Donnell, J. (1971). Methlyphenidate problems (cont.) (third letter). *The New England Journal of Medicine, 285*(17), 970.

Ohan, J. L., & Johnston, C. (2005). Gender Appropriateness of Symptom Criteria for Attention-Deficit/Hyperactivity Disorder, Oppositional-Defiant Disorder, and Conduct Disorder. [References]. *Child Psychiatry & Human Development, 35*(4), 359–381.

Parens, E., & Johnston, J. (2009). Facts, values, and Attention-Deficit Hyperactivity Disorder (ADHD): an update on the controversies. *Child Adolesc Psychiatry Ment Health, 3*(1), 1.

Pastor, P. N., & Reuben, C. A. (2005). Racial and Ethnic Differences in ADHD and LD in Young School-Age Children: Parental Reports in the National Health Interview Survey. *Public Health Reports, 120*(July-August), 383–392.

Pelham, W. E., Foster, E. M., & Robb, J. A. (2007). The economic impact of attention-deficit/hyperactivity disorder in children and adolescents. *Ambul Pediatr, 7*(1 Suppl), 121–131.

Peppercorn, J., Blood, E., Winer, E., & Partridge, A. (2007). Association between pharmaceutical involvement and outcomes in breast cancer clinical trials. *Cancer, 109*(7), 1239–1246.

President's Commission on Special Education (2002). *A New Era: Revitalizing Special Education for Children and Their Families.* Jessup, MD: U.S. Department of Education, Office of Special Education and Rehabilitative Services.

Purdie, N., Hattie, J., & Carroll, A. (2002). A review of the research on interventions for attention deficit hyperactivity disorder: what works best? *Review of Educational Research, 72*(1), 61–99.

Quinn, P. O. (2005). Treating Adolescent Girls and Women With ADHD: Gender-Specific Issues. [References]. *Journal of Clinical Psychology, 61*(5), 579–587.

Rapp, M. S. (1971). Methylphenidate problems (cont.) (first letter). *The New England Journal of Medicine, 285*(17), 970.

Renstrom, R. (1976). The teacher and the social worker in stimulant drug treatment of hyperactive children. *School Review, 85*(1), 97–108.

Robison, L. M., Sclar, D. A., & Skaer, T. L. (2005). Trends in ADHD and stimulant use among adults: 1995–2002. *Psychiatric Services, 56*(12), 1497.

Robison, L. M., Sclar, D. A., Skaer, T. L., & Galin, R. S. (1999). National trends in the prevalence of attention-deficit/hyperactivity disorder and the prescribing of methylphenidate among school-age children: 1990–1995. *Clinical Pediatrics, 38*(4), 209–217.

Rouse, J. (1987). *Knowledge and Power: Toward a Political Philosophy of Science.* Ithaca, NY: Cornell University Press.

Rowland, A. S., Lesesne, C. A., & Abramowitz, A. J. (2002). The epidemiology of attention-deficit/hyperactivity disorder (ADHD): a public health view. *Mental Retardation and Developmental Disabilities, 8,* 162–170.

Sax, L., & Kautz, K. J. (2003). Who first suggests the diagnosis of attention-deficit/hyperactivity disorder? *Annals of Family Medicine, 1*(3), 171–174.

Schneider, H., & Eisenberg, D. (2006). Who receives a diagnosis of attention-deficit/hyperactivity disorder in the United States elementary school population? *Pediatrics, 117*(4), e601–e609.

Schwartz, M. L., Pizzo, S. V., McKee, P. A. (1971). Minimal brain dysfunction and methylphenidate (letter). *The New England Journal of Medicine, 285*(5), 293.

Singh, I. (2005). Will the "real boy" please behave: Dosing dilemmas for parents of boys with ADHD. *The American Journal of Bioethics, 5*(3), 34–47.

Sonuga-Barke, E. J. S., Dalen, L., & Remington, B. (2003). Do executive deficits and delay aversion make independent contributions to preschool attention-deficit/hyperactivity disorder symptoms? *Journal of the American Academy of Child and Adolescent Psychiatry, 42*(11), 1335–1342.

Stevens, J., Harman, J. S., & Kelleher, K. J. (2005). Race/ethnicity and insurance status as factors associated with ADHD treatment patterns. *Journal of Child and Adolescent Psychopharmacology, 15*(1), 88–96.

Subcommittee on Education Reform, Committee on Education and the Workforce (2002): *Rethinking Special Education: How to Reform the Individuals with Disabilities Education Act.* Washington, D.C.: House of Representatives, One Hundred Seventh Congress.

Swing, E. L., Gentile, D. A., Anderson, C. A., & Walsh, D. A. (2010). Television and video game exposure and the development of attention problems. *Pediatrics, 126*(2), 214–221.

U.S. Department of Education, Office of Special Education and Rehabilitative Services, Office of Special Education Programs (2006). *Teaching children with attention deficit hyperactivity disorder: Instructional strategies and practices.* Washington, D.C.

U.S. Department of Health and Human Services (2000). *Healthy People 2010: Understanding and Improving Health,* 2nd ed. Washington, D.C.: U.S. Government Printing Office.

U.S. Department of Health and Human Services. (2010). Healthy People 2020: Topics and Objectives: Mental Health and Mental Disorders Retrieved January 17, 2011, from http://www.healthypeople.gov/2020/topicsobjectives2020/overview.aspx?topicid=28

Van Acker, R., Boreson, L., Frankenberger, W., O'Donnell, D., Keniston, A., Rau, R., et al. (2002). *Students with disabilities in general education classrooms: Their experiences and impact*: University of Wisconsin—Eau Claire, University of Illinois at Chicago, Wisconsin Department of Public Instruction.

Wikler, A., Dixon, J. F., & Parker, J. B. (1970). Brain function in problem children and controls: psychometric, neurological, and electroencephalographic comparisons. *American Journal of Psychiatry, 127*(5), 634–645.

Willey, R. F. (1971). Abuse of methylphenidate (Ritalin) (letter). *The New England Journal of Medicine, 285,* 464.

Woodruff, T. J., Axelrad, D. A., Kyle, A. D., Nweke, O., Miller, G. G., & Hurley, B. J. (2004). Trends in environmentally related childhood illnesses. *Pediatrics, 113*(4), 1133–1140.

Wright, J. (1995). Attention-deficit hyperactivity disorder: a school-based evaluation manual. Retrieved January 15, 2007, from http://www.interventioncentral.org

Xu, C., Reid, R., & Steckelberg, A. (2002). Technology applications for children with ADHD: assessing the empirical support. *Education and Treatment of Children, 25*(2), 224–248.

Zalecki, C. A., & Hinshaw, S. P. (2004). Overt and Relational Aggression in Girls With Attention Deficit Hyperactivity Disorder. [References]. *Journal of Clinical Child and Adolescent Psychology, 33*(1), 125–137.

Zito, J. M. (2000). Pharmacoepidemiology of methylphenidate and other medications for the treatment of ADHD, in R. W. Manderscheid & M. J. Henderson (Eds.) *Mental Health, United States, 2000.* Substance Abuse and Mental Health Services Administration, Report No. SMA-01-3537, Rockville, MD, 113–119.

Zoler, M. L. (2010). Prevalence of ADHD in U.S. youths reached 9.5% in 2007–2008. *Internal Medicine News Digital Network.* Retrieved January 27, 2011, from http://www.internalmedicinenews.com/index.php?id=495&cHash=071010&tx_ttnews[tt_news]=18359

NOTES

1. According to Latour's actor-network theory, a scientific fact, model, or paradigm is held in place not because is it "true," but because it has a broader network of associations—with other facts, existing literature, available tools, people's needs—than an alternative that is "false." In Latour's view, establishing these networks is the activity of science; cognitive factors considered apart from these activities are largely unnecessary in establishing facts. He argues that the activity of convincing others of the strength of one's findings cannot be distinguished from the activity of recruiting them as allies in one's cause. If one finding is supported by a bigger laboratory, more expensive and sophisticated tools, more funding, more allies, more publications, and so forth (i.e., the finding has more nodes in its network), that finding, rather than one with fewer nodes, will be considered a fact. Further, once a strong network is in place, dissent becomes difficult and expensive. In Latour's view, then, "construction of facts" such as those about the existence, definition, and treatment of ADHD is a "collective process" (Latour, 1987, 29). Latour's is not simply a "social construction" view, however. In part, this is because social constructionist views tend to pit society and science against one another, followed by the claim that social factors are primary in knowledge formation. Latour, instead, rejects the dichotomization of scientific and social, rational and irrational, subjective and objective, in favor of his account of activities and strengths. Actor-network theory is also differentiated from social constructionist views in that whatever is being investigated will resist some manipulations and yield to others. This means that not anything goes—facts must be answerable to the responses of

people, but they must also be answerable to empirical constraints. In more Latourian language, the cooperation of the various "actants"—those "some-things" (what would ordinarily be called people or things under investigation) represented and reshaped in scientific discourse—is required to establish the networks, along with the investigator's active forging of links with the literature and with human "allies."

2. The argument does not depend on accepting Latour's views, however. Readers are welcome to consider actor-network theory a metaphor for the complex interactions traced in the chapter; I describe a key interaction—the entrance of social values into the sciences of ADHD—in more analytic terms in Chapter 4.
3. I necessarily discuss the role of ADHD-diagnosable individuals and parents in this chapter, but its centrality requires separate treatment as well, in Chapter 5.
4. It is impossible to cleanly separate these controversies, which relate primarily to views expressed by organized or quasi-organized groups concerning the ramifications of pragmatic, sociopolitical, and ethical decisions *on* ADHD-diagnosable individuals from those expressed *by* those individuals, but I roughly save the latter for Chapter 5.
5. Section 504 is a civil rights law named for a section of the Rehabilitation Act of 1973. It guarantees nondiscrimination by federally funded entities such as public schools, but, unlike regulations governing special education, it does not provide additional funding to the schools.
6. Comorbidity, or concomitant diagnosis, is the rule rather than the exception for ADHD-diagnosable individuals (*see* Chapter 1).
7. Children classified in the OHI category generally spend much of their day in general classrooms, as do those with diagnosed specific learning disabilities; those designated emotionally disturbed typically spend less time in regular classrooms (Education, 2002, Tables 1–7).
8. Other diagnoses among those that qualify under the "other health impairment" category are diabetes, epilepsy, and heart disease.
9. This point raises the contentious issue of whether the federal government fulfills its funding commitments, but that issue goes too far afield.
10. National reports do not subdivide the general categories according to specific diagnoses of the children so classified, but state reports sometimes do. For example, in one school district in Wisconsin, 87.5% of those eligible for special education in the OHI category had ADHD (Van Acker et al., 2002).
11. In 2002, 0.6% of the school-age population (ages 6–21 years) received special education services under the OHI category (Education, 2002). If ADHD diagnosability is estimated at a conservative 5%, and about 90% of those receiving OHI services have ADHD (Van Acker et al., 2002), then about 10% of those who have ADHD receive special education services under the OHI category. The number of those in the specific learning disability and emotional disturbance categories who have ADHD cannot be estimated from the information readily available.

12. Parents are not a uniform class. For example, parental gender, place of birth (United States or not), state of residence, race, and family income all correlate with differences in rates of their children's' diagnosis (Schneider & Eisenberg, 2006). I discuss some of these differences in the second section of Chapter 2. I also consider complex and individualized aspects of parental decisions regarding their children in Chapter 5.
13. A survey asked physicians in several specialties who had first suggested that a child might "have" ADHD. The clinicians estimated that 52% of the first suggestions were by school personnel (46% by teachers), 30% by parents, and 14% by clinicians. The remainder represented a variety of other sources (Sax & Kautz, 2003).
14. Children's attitudes toward diagnosis and treatment have not been well studied (Bastiaansen, Koot, Ferdinand, & Verhulst, 2004), although Ilina Singh's work, discussed in Chapter 5, is beginning to address this gap.
15. Available data on psychologists' involvement in ADHD treatment is not comparable in the level of detail available for physicians' involvement. However, despite the fact that there is support for some forms of behavior therapy in the literature, the trend is toward medication and away from psychotherapy (Leslie & Wolraich, 2007).
16. Efficacy was judged by the cost to "normalize" a child's SNAP scores. SNAP is a checklist of symptoms of ADHD, oppositional defiant disorder, and other childhood mental disorders that are part of ADHD's differential diagnosis. To complete the SNAP, parents and teachers rate the child on such items as "Has difficulty attending to a group classroom activity or discussion (Response choices: Not at all/Just a little/Quite a bit/Very much)." "Normalization" means that a previously ADHD-diagnosable child's ratings are, following or under treatment, within age-group norms. Complications concerning this definition of efficacy, and concerning treatment preferences, are discussed in Chapters 4 and 5.
17. This topic is covered in more detail in Chapter 4.
18. *But see* Chapter 5 regarding destigmatization vs. forms of intolerance that are reinforced by current views of ADHD.
19. From 1980 to 1987, ADHD's precursor category, ADD, was in use, and adult ADHD was not well recognized; hence, the group's acronym. (http://www.chadd.org/Content/CHADD/AboutCHADD/Mission/default.htm; accessed February 16, 2007).
20. http://www.help4adhd.org/en/about/myths. Accessed February 17, 2007.
21. CHADD's Income and Expenditures (2008–2009), Accessed October 3, 2010 from http://www.chadd.org/AM/Template.cfm?Section=Reports1&Template=/CM/ContentDisplay.cfm&ContentID=13230.
22. Drug company research funding data are proprietary and so not included here.
23. There is an important distinction between laboratory "efficacy" and "effectiveness" in the social environment.

24. Currently, 5 million people are taking prescription medication for ADHD (more have been diagnosed). However, if Biederman et al. are correct in their estimate of ADHD prevalence (approximately 10% in children and adolescents, 5% in adults; Biederman & Faraone, 2005), the figure should be about 17.5 million, assuming all were prescribed medication and those aged 70 years and older opted out of the diagnosis.
25. Alternatively, many of those undiagnosed might happily embrace the diagnosis but have not had access to a clinician attentive to the possibility; this possibility is addressed under "Equity."
26. Accessed December 10, 2007 from http://www.nami.org/Content/NavigationMenu/Inform_Yourself/About_NAMI/About_NAMI.htm.
27. Only 10% of U.S. clinical trials of drugs are supported by the NIH; most of the additional support is provided by drug companies (Angell, 2004).
28. CHADD's primary policy advocacy, according to its web site, concerns IDEA (*see* "Education, special education," above), which it addresses through the Children's Behavioral Alliance (a coalition organized by CHADD). The Children's Behavioral Alliance does have school-based membership (the National Association of School Psychologists and the School Social Work Association of America), but no education groups per se.
29. Burns is concerned about special education labeling in general, including but not limited to the ADHD diagnosis. He also questions the validity of most ADHD diagnoses (personal communication).
30. In 2002, the percentages of students of each racial/ethnic group (American Indian/Alaskan Native, Asian/Pacific Islander, Black [not Hispanic], Hispanic, and White [not Hispanic]) placed in these categories, were (2002): Other health impairment: 5.0, 4.8, 5.1, 3.6, and 8.0, respectively; and Emotional disorders: 7.9, 4.7, 11.3, 4.9, 7.9, respectively.

4 FEEDBACK: VALUES IN ADHD SCIENCE

Philosophers, historians, and sociologists have long since refuted the idea that science is free of social influence. Yet the ideal of scientific objectivity persists. According to this ideal, although social values and interests often sway a scientist's choice of projects—by providing more funding for research that's clearly useful, for example—the methodology and conclusions of science should (and usually do) resist the potentially biasing effects of social influence. When true to this ideal, science stands apart from the sociopolitical morass and can therefore be called in as a neutral judge on well-studied issues. I want not to be taken wrong: I think that science *is* a crucial touchstone for sociopolitical decisions, including decisions about how best to respond to the difficulties of ADHD-diagnosable individuals. However, the reason for this is not that science is value free.

One reason we might suspect that the sciences that study ADHD would violate the ideal is that their object of inquiry—"ADHD"—has values embedded in its definition. The concept of "disorder" has negative connotations, as do the specific symptoms that define ADHD.[1] Symptoms such as "fails to give close attention to details or makes careless mistakes in schoolwork, work, or other activities," and "loses things necessary for tasks or activities" denote behaviors that violate social norms (American Psychiatric Association, 2000, 92–93). An ADHD diagnosis also requires impairment in (American Psychiatric Association, 2000) or negative impact on (American Psychiatric Association, 2013) social, academic, or occupational activities. Because ADHD is by definition undesirable in these and other ways, whatever scientists find when they study ADHD necessarily leaves this valence negative—that is, whatever refinements are made in the scientific understanding of ADHD, "impairment" or negative impact—and therefore "having" ADHD—will still be undesirable.

But that does not necessarily mean that the value valence colors the refinements of the concept, such as new information about the genetics, neurophysiology, or treatment of ADHD.[2] According to the persisting ideal, scientists can study a value-valenced object of inquiry impartially, such that social norms, interests, and other values do not influence their conclusions. To what extent do the sciences that study ADHD meet this ideal? Consider the following conclusions, representing a range of studies of ADHD:

> ...our meta-analyses suggest that DRD4 is a susceptibility gene for ADHD (Faraone, Doyle, Mick, & Biederman, 2001, 1055).
> ...these results suggest that children with ADHD (or even those at a subthreshold diagnostic level) will benefit from behavioral strategies that address their symptoms of ADHD and help them to achieve to their potential in the classroom (Barry, Lyman, & Klinger, 2002, 279).
> ...studies that generate culturally appropriate approaches to educating African-American parents about the causes and treatment alternatives for ADHD may well be important in removing the barriers to seeking help for their children (Bussing, Gary, Mills, & Garvan, 2003, 573).

> In stimulant-responsive young children with ADHD without learning and conduct disorders, there is no support for academic assistance and psychotherapy to enhance academic achievement or emotional adjustment (Hechtman, et al., 2004, 812).

> ...our findings suggest that carefully monitored medication treatment, although not quite as effective as the combination of medication and behavioral treatment, is likely to be more cost-effective in routine treatment for children with ADHD, particularly those without comorbid conduct disorders (Jensen et al., 2005, 1635).

Do the needs and interests of clinicians, parents, teachers, industry, government, and others in venues discussed in earlier chapters influence these conclusions? If the conclusions are "influenced," in what sense is that the case? This chapter argues that social values, needs, and interests strongly influence the practice and conclusions of the ADHD sciences. To do this, it re-examines scientists' practices and data analyses in the light of the social context described in the past several chapters.[3] Doing so will show what the social influence is and how it arises. (Other chapters explore ways in which the sciences, in turn, alter social practice and concepts.) The influence is only sometimes caused by overt bias in favor of some interest. Pervasively, though, trends in what aspects of ADHD are studied and connotations of language and concepts used to interpret data reinforce the negative connotations of ADHD. Common research methodologies also directly and indirectly sharpen the value valence, especially by way of dichotomizing ADHD from "normal." These observations neither debunk ADHD science nor idolize it. Instead, they explain where the influence of social values and interests enters the sciences that study ADHD and how it is made to stick.

Containable Bias

A study is overtly biased when a researcher designs a study or manipulates data to prove a predetermined point. Research funded by the pharmaceutical industry is often suspected of bias, given the lucrative market for ADHD interventions. Yet, despite the fact that various parties have strong interests in particular results, studies funded by drug companies are often well designed. Competing interests of scientists, journal editors, and the public in objective, unbiased research usually protect against overt bias in individual studies. Several analyses show, however, that industry-sponsored clinical trials are more likely to give favorable results for the sponsor's product than are similar studies not supported by industry (Kelly et al., 2006; Lexchin, Bero, Djulbegovic, & Clark, 2003; Melander, Ahlqvist-Rastad, Meijer, & Beermann, 2004; Peppercorn, Blood, Winer, & Partridge, 2007). One explanation for this phenomenon is publication bias: Sponsors suppress publication of unfavorable results (Krimsky, 2003; Lemmens, 2004). This biases the literature by painting an overly rosy picture of a product's efficacy. Another explanation is that study designs are innocuously biased: Positive results for the company predominate because the sponsor only pays to test products that prior research suggests are likely to get favorable results (Fries & Krishnan, 2004). This strategy is "innocuous" as long as the prior research included a search for alternative strategies and as long as prior studies seriously attempted to disprove the hoped-for outcome. Depending on the degree of publication bias and whether study design truly is innocuous, industry sponsorship—or other self-interested support or perspective—may or may not result in overt bias in individual articles or the literature as a whole.

Even if bias is not overt in the sense given above, individual studies may not so subtly examine issues in a way that slants results in the authors' or sponsors' favor. For example, prominent psychopharmacologist Joseph Biederman and psychiatrist Stephen Faraone, who frequently publish in top-tier journals in their fields, published a minor article titled "The Effects of Attention-Deficit/Hyperactivity Disorder on Employment and Household Income" in the online journal *Medscape Today* (Biederman & Faraone, 2006, unpaginated). The article compares responses of 500 ADHD-diagnosed adults and 501 age- and gender-matched controls to a telephone survey. Among other questions, respondents were asked their age, educational attainment, and household income. The conclusion of the study was that those who had ADHD had lower household income, on average, than those without ADHD, with a resulting loss to the U.S. economy of $67 billion to $116 billion annually. The central bias of the article is hinted at in the phrase "on average." The authors acknowledge that the reported lower income is simply assumed to result from the respondents' ADHD *per se*, and they note that one unexamined possibility is that the lower income relates more directly to comorbid learning disability than to ADHD. Yet relevant alternatives (comorbid disorders or other important differences among ADHD-diagnosed individuals, individual preference and/or satisfaction in jobs, etc.) are unexplored, and the conclusion is stated flatly: "Decreased individual income among adults with ADHD contributes to substantial loss in US workforce productivity." One cannot be sure without exploring the alternatives, but it may be that the study can maintain its strong conclusion only by avoiding pertinent questions. It is hard to resist the interpretation that the avoidance was purposeful: Shire Pharmaceuticals, maker of Adderall, a commonly prescribed ADHD medication, sponsored the study, and both authors report research support from multiple drug companies, service on several drug companies' speakers' bureaus, and positions on drug company advisory boards.

But scientists and laypeople alike know that they should be alert to potentially biasing influences of industry sponsorship or ideological viewpoints. Peer review and research ethics policies can in principle detect and constrain overt and unsubtle bias. But even when observing these policies does weed out overt and unsubtle bias, social influence still pervades ADHD science. The subtler influences of social needs and interests are harder to identify, but it is these influences that are the norm.

Investigative Trends

The pharmaceutical industry's needs and interests have influenced the sciences of ADHD even without overt bias in individual articles. One way in which this is the case is that the large number of sponsored studies contributes to the direction—and the conclusions—of research. This section details how that happens. But the point is hardly unique to industry-sponsored research. Other trends in research also create a pattern of accumulations and gaps in knowledge, shaping current understanding of ADHD (Furman, 2008). For example, a biological rather than environmental or psychosocial orientation dominates ADHD research, and short-term studies greatly outweigh long-term. Overall, the values that drive interest or disinterest in particular areas of inquiry color the scientific understanding of ADHD—but this point will be clearer with some detailed examples in hand.

That investigative trends shape the *direction* of research is obvious. In fact, to a large extent investigative trends *are* the direction of research, although research done outside the mainstream also contributes. But the trends also shape the *conclusions* of the research. Higher-level trends—for example, that ADHD is a relevant object of inquiry—quite clearly affect the body of scientific knowledge. (We wouldn't know much about ADHD if we didn't study it.) At this level, where the categories worthy of investigation are predefined, guiding the research of groups of investigators, and enabling comparison of data among investigators, trends function much like Kuhnian paradigms (Kuhn, 1996 [1962]). Like Kuhn's paradigms, the concept "ADHD" structures research for scientists who study it by establishing basic assumptions, such as using the *Diagnostic and Statistical Manual of Mental Disorders* (DSM) (American Psychiatric Association, 2000; American Psychiatric Association, 2013) criteria for selecting research subjects; criteria for data interpretation, such as knowledge of typical mental function, brain structure, and behavior; and appropriate research methodologies. Such criteria strongly influence what comes to be known about ADHD and ADHD-associated phenomena.

Similarly, trends within ADHD research shape ADHD knowledge. For example, we have more detail about response to specific drugs than we do about the effects of environment on symptom appearance or severity, simply because the former has been studied more intensively. Ideally, scientific conclusions are not moderated by the "bulk of the evidence"—the cumulative result of a trend—but by other evidentiary considerations.[4] Yet, although the inference is not scientifically ideal, available evidence is sometimes claimed to outweigh absent (as opposed to negative) evidence. For example, neuroscientists hypothesize that perturbations in the manufacture, uptake, and distribution of neurotransmitters (the "chemical messengers" of the brain, such as dopamine, serotonin, and norepinephrine) underlie many symptoms of mental illness and disorders. In the case of ADHD, the role of dopamine has received the most study, because methylphenidate (Ritalin) and other stimulants have long been known to reduce ADHD symptoms, and they also, via multiple mechanisms, increase the availability and uptake of dopamine in the brain (Wilens, 2008). But other studies—and the efficacy of drugs that target alternate pathways, such as atomoxetine (Strattera) and buproprion (Wellbutrin)—have suggested that the neurotransmitters norepinephrine and serotonin might be involved as well (Mayes, Bagwell, & Erkulwater, 2009; Oades, 2007; Tripp & Wickens, 2009). The predominance of dopamine research has allowed some authors to draw (in part) on bulk-of-the-evidence arguments to make a case for dopamine's involvement in ADHD etiology. For example, in supporting their theory that dysfunction in the brain's dopamine system explains all symptoms of hyperactive/impulsive-type ADHD, Sagvolden et al. write, "...the *majority of* findings from a variety of research fields seem to converge on dopamine in the etiology of ADHD..." (Sagvolden, Aase, Johansen, & Russell, 2005, 409, emphasis added). But a commentator points out that contending hypotheses have been downgraded by default. It is true, she agrees, that the bulk of the evidence favors dopamine, "...but ADHD research has been excessively biased towards dopamine investigation, and the few studies that have investigated the involvement of other neurotransmitters have been positive" (Rubia, 2005, 440). Despite the positive evidence they cite, Rubia argues, Sagvolden et al. should not make a definitive claim for their dopamine hypothesis, as other viable hypotheses have not received adequate study.

The long-term "excessive bias" Rubia mentions has had a practical result: a 30+-year emphasis on stimulant therapy for ADHD. This approach has many proponents and successes, but it has left other options underexplored—not only research concerning other medications, which have received more attention in the past decade, but also non-drug therapy. A practical result of scientific study is not identical to the "scientific conclusion" of a specific article, a meta-analysis, or the consensus in a field. Yet the "practical result" of the emphasis promotes a view of ADHD that foregrounds its (typical) responsiveness to stimulant medication. To deny the effect of this and other investigative trends on scientists' data interpretations, methodologies, requests for funding, clinical recommendations, and other aspects of scientific practice, is to argue that a field of clinical researchers can be somehow disengaged from effects of clinical context on their thought. ADHD researchers are not disengaged. These trends shape aggregate scientific knowledge of ADHD.

More generally in the intervention literature, articles on pharmacotherapy outnumber those on behavior therapy by approximately 10:1 and outnumber those on academic intervention by about 7:1.[5] The de-emphasis on academic interventions has been noted since the early 1990s, which means the gap reaches into the 1980s. In the early 1990s, there was a push from parents to make ADHD diagnosis (then often known by the earlier name "attention deficit disorder" or ADD) an explicit criterion of eligibility for special education programs in the schools. To help assess the need for this change, the U.S. Department of Education asked the Chesapeake Institute of Washington, D.C., to prepare a report on current practice in identification and management of the disorder in the school setting. The Institute authors found that there was only a limited database from which they could draw conclusions:

> The generalizability and interpretation of the research on educational characteristics of children with ADD is limited by a number of factors. First, since most of the research was conducted and reported from a mental health perspective and used clinical rather than school-based samples, there is less evidence available [for effective school-based assessment and intervention strategies] than might be expected, given that the initial literature base contained over a thousand articles[6]... This limits the research base in the following ways. First, information on educational characteristics is rarely reported, which narrows the literature base to about 90 articles. Second, when this literature is narrowed further on the basis of type of educational characteristic and type of sample, there is very little replication of studies (Chesapeake Institute, 1993, 23–24 [McKinney et al.]).

The small number of studies and dearth of replications made any data analysis tenuous, even when practices showed promise. Yet this trend has not changed in intervening years. In addition, there are trends and gaps within the education literature. The editor of a special issue of the *Journal of Attention Disorders* focusing on school-based treatment of ADHD noted that recent and current literature focuses on individual interventions and interventions in primary school settings (Evans, 2005). In contrast, he writes, school-wide interventions are relatively unexplored, as are school-based treatments for those in junior high and high schools.

More generally still, the research emphasis has been on conceiving and investigating ADHD as a biological dysfunction (Mayes et al., 2009; *see also* Chapters 1 and 2). Typical targets of current research include ADHD's genetics, its underlying neural and chemical structures, and intervention with targeted medications. Such foci are important for a full understanding of ADHD—like any trait or behavior, ADHD-associated phenomena involve biological activity. But the complexity of ADHD as a phenomenon argues that research trends have been too narrowly focused. In particular, ADHD is also a social phenomenon. The network of social structures, relationships, and expectations in which ADHD-diagnosable individuals find themselves is relevant to what they do and how their actions are perceived and evaluated. In addition, positive studies exist in the behavior therapy and school psychology literature (DuPaul, 2007; Pelham & Fabiano, 2008), suggesting that aspects of social structures and interactions, as well as educational approaches, could potentially be manipulated for ADHD-diagnosable individuals' benefit. With this broader perspective in mind, it seems reasonable that non–biologically oriented sciences could contribute more to the understanding of ADHD than they do at present. No guarantee exists that shifting the balance of research would be fruitful, yet it remains the case that the current understanding of ADHD has been shaped in part by what is not known about it.

In Chapter 3, I argued that our current understanding of ADHD has derived value valence from the practices, needs, and interests of parents, clinicians, teachers, employers, the pharmaceutical industry, and others. Investigative trends also color the way ADHD is understood, expressing and reinforcing a package of values congruent with many of those discussed earlier. For example, the emphasis on biologically oriented research helps structure current models of ADHD in accord with the needs and interests of medicine and its allied fields—that is, biomedical science studies factors that biomedicine is poised to address. Foci within the biomedical literature—on ADHD as a dysfunction in the individual, on intervening at the level of the individual, on pharmacological approaches that lend themselves to clinical efficiency and short-term behavioral control—are consistent not only with medicine, but also with many of the values that drive concern about ADHD in other venues. Studying intervention at the individual level fits the investigative results to the capabilities of medicine (Krimsky, 2003, 224). Pharmacological approaches address drug company interests; in contrast, studies of environmental contributions to ADHD symptomatology, whether stresses and inflexible social structures or environmental toxins, would provide few opportunities for product development (Krimsky, 2003, 180). Emphasis on short-term behavioral control addresses immediate (although not necessarily the long-term) needs and interests of teachers, parents, and many ADHD-diagnosable individuals. On a higher level, the investigation of ADHD itself marks an investigative trend within the study of mental function and dysfunction. Other aspects of function, departures from "normal," or different symptom complexes might have been studied, but ADHD was among the phenomena identified as socially or medically important. By emphasizing topics consistent with particular values, current investigative trends shape the concept of ADHD in accord with those values.

Deeper Embedding: What Questions? What Assumptions?

The emphases and omissions of investigative trends have broad-strokes influence on science. But these do not necessarily affect the conclusions of individual studies: no matter what the topic, studies can in principle be carried out and interpreted objectively, without introducing social values—or so the argument goes. A close look, however, shows that social values commonly valence the conclusions of individual studies. What's more, the practice of science itself favors certain types of conclusions. These influences are embedded in the current understanding of ADHD.

The influence of values on the sciences of ADHD is one instance in a general pattern. For example, Gannett (2001) argues that population geneticists incorporate racist values in scientific conclusions when they look for genetic differences among populations. This does not mean that the population geneticists are themselves racists—instead, some common assumptions are. When this goes unrecognized (or is recognized but not corrected), the assumptions valence data interpretation. The population geneticists argue that their work is protected from racism because they simply seek patterns in the genome, independent of social context or values; pattern-seeking is a matter of reading and counting DNA sequences—objective, value-free activities. But Gannett counters that more is needed for data interpretation. To recognize the patterns in the DNA sequences, the scientists must focus on a particular part of the genome—that is, they must identify genes of interest. To say that a genetic effect causes differences in a trait (associated traits often being what make a gene interesting), the models must also assume that there is no variation in the environment. Otherwise, the contribution of the genes to variation in traits cannot be detected. These assumptions mean that racist values may privilege interest in certain traits and genes and that the contributions of racist structures in society (the environment) to any given trait may be ignored. For these reasons, cultural meanings may become embedded in the conclusions of the science. In Gannett's words,

> It is not nature that determines distinctions like that between "fundamental" and "superficial" characteristics; it is not nature that encourages biologists to relegate non-genetic causal factors to the necessary

background against which genes exert their effects; it is not nature that leads geneticists to investigate DNA differences associated with some physiological or behavioral differences and not others...The persistence of racist structures in society means not only that "facts" about group DNA differences can be "misused" to racist ends but that such "facts" will incorporate those cultural meanings that attach to human differences (S491–S492).

In this instance, then, values become embedded in conclusions of individual articles, as well as a field of study, via what scientists choose to study and by the assumptions of their analyses.

Longino (1990) highlights the role of background assumptions as a source of values in science, arguing that value-valenced assumptions are sometimes used to justify scientific conclusions. This is a special case of her more general claim that some assumptions (value valenced or not) are needed to fill in the gaps between what someone observes and what s/he hypothesizes about the observations. Perhaps someone observes a broken vase, for example. Vases can break in many ways—among them, sudden winds, cold snaps, leaping cats, wagging tails, and rambunctious toddlers. The simple observation "broken vase" *underdetermines* the theory that explains the observation: the observer needs additional evidence to determine the cause. But what evidence? Different observers can bring different assumptions to their reasoning: One might assume that the window is easy to open, another that thermostats are unreliable. One might be of the mind that pets are nuisances, and another think that children wreak havoc. Such background assumptions favor one hypothesis over by directing the observer's attention toward particular types of evidence. One observer might note the Duplos on the floor and ignore the pet hair, concluding that a toddler was the culprit. Another might close the window against the wind but ignore the still-frigid air.

The investigation would not need to end with the initial observation and gathering of evidence, of course. If there were need to determine the cause of the broken vase with certainty, the observer could investigate his/her own assumptions, empirically confirming their truth or falsity. After the observer checked out all reasonable hypotheses (the window, the thermostat, pet or child behavior, and others), their "research" might favor new hypotheses and/or suggest additional evidence. In more complex settings, such as scientific research on complex problems, Longino argues that there will come a point at which the researcher must stop investigating. At that point, a value-valenced assumption can guide data interpretation without researchers' awareness.

This arguably occurs in the case Gannett describes—the scientists involved may simply not see that, for example, thinking of certain forms of intelligence as worthy of study assumes that those forms are *good* or *important* in some way—that is, a value is attributed to a trait and that value becomes embedded in the science that seeks knowledge of the trait. In this way, scientists may often choose a hypothesis that serves a particular value-valenced criterion or need. Importantly, some of the values will be the epistemic values of science—the *simpler* hypothesis will be favored, or the one that better *coheres* with other data (*see* Chapter 2). But other such values will be contextual—the social needs and interests that emphasize such criteria as utility or ethical principles. Many such assumptions pervade the sciences of ADHD; assumptions about desirable forms of attention, behavior, intelligence, and achievement direct scientists' attention and interpretations toward particular conclusions. We can see this at work in the language of scientific interpretation.

Deeper Embedding: Language and Context

When we use language, we bring a lifetime of associations to each word, concept, or phrase. For me, the word, "water" conjures up the drinking fountain in Heller Hall, sauna steam, sea-sickness, lake swims, the YMCA's chlorinated pool (etc., etc.) and—more abstractly, because I've never seen two "hydrogens" or an "oxygen"—water's chemical composition. To you, "water" connotes something a little different, because of the multitude of associations you bring to the term—its context. When scientists use language in interpreting their data, some words are highly technical and decontextualized—but not all. The rich connotations of the latter can valence scientific conclusions.

Putnam (2002) discusses a class of words that consistently carries important connotations, the dual-use "thick ethical terms." One use is *description* of an object, person, event, or phenomenon; the other is *prescription* of a proper attitude toward that object, person, event, or phenomenon. The key, however, is that the dual use is *simultaneous*—when using such a term, one necessarily applies both descriptive and prescriptive elements of the word, although the relative emphasis on description or prescription can vary with context. To use the word "cruel," for example, I might list specific acts of a despot and call them cruel (emphasizing the descriptive sense); or I might judge the despot's character "cruel" (with relatively more normative intent). In either case, to fully understand the term, my audience needs to understand both the normative and the descriptive content. More generally, hearers/readers need to recognize that the evaluative content persists even when speakers/writers use thick ethical terms as if the evaluative content had been excised. Thick ethical terms appear ubiquitously in the scientific literature concerning ADHD; despite clinical denotations, evaluative content persists in words such as "abnormal," "disorder," "dysfunction," "deficiency," "deficit," "inattention," "hyperactivity," "impulsivity," and their positively valenced converses. Scientists, intentionally or unintentionally, express values when they use these terms.

Often, technical scientific language is highly decontextualized. When the terms refer to equipment or phenomena that are known more or less exclusively by a small group of scientists with advanced training in a field, the opportunities for contextualization are fewer and those for complete and detailed description are greater. For example, the following sentence occurs in a paper that reported electroencephalogram (EEG) results, recorded while ADHD-diagnosed children completed a computerized "stop task": "A main effect revealed N2 amplitude was larger across the scalp for FI than SI trials, although within the midlateral comparisons, the difference showed a midline > lateral sites effect that was maximal in the central region" (Dimoska, Johnstone, Barry, & Clarke, 2003, 1349). This sentence mentions a statistical analysis (main effect), a component of the EEG record (N2 amplitude), abbreviations for variations in the testing protocol (FI and SI trials), and variation in effects among anatomical landmarks (midlateral, midline, lateral, central). This kind of reporting is typical, especially, of the "Results" sections of scientific articles. By virtue of its lack of context, it is relatively value-neutral, although even here values are embedded in the interest in whatever is being described, the operationalization chosen, and in the criteria for choosing subgroups. This point explains why the concept of "difference" between groups is only *relatively* value-free in the clinical sciences, compared with attributions of "dysfunction" and the rest (*see also* Fig. 4.1).

But scientific articles do not stop with basic reporting of results. Scientists also want colleagues and other readers to interpret their results in particular ways—they want it to be clear how their observations support or disagree with other papers in the field, how their paper contributes to knowledge of their subject matter, or ways it suggests practical solutions to problems relevant to their subject matter. In short, they want readers to agree with conclusions they believe the data corroborate. This push toward practical implementation is pronounced in clinical science, which prizes clinical significance. The papers typically have "Introduction" and "Discussion" sections that undertake this work. In these sections, connotation and context are likely to be important to the scientists' goals—and may contribute to valencing the paper's conclusions.

One conclusion of Dimoska et al.'s EEG study is that ADHD-diagnosed children are slower to inhibit their reactions to stimuli than are non-ADHD children. In the "stop task" the children performed in that study, for example, the children were set a "primary task" of reacting to a "T" or an "O" appearing on a computer screen by pressing "T" or "O," respectively, on a keyboard. Sometimes, though, a tone heard through headphones closely followed the appearance of the letter; when this happened, the child was supposed to refrain from pressing the letter. The 13 ADHD-diagnosed children took, on average, 100 msec longer than the 13 non-ADHD children to respond to the stop signal. The EEG recording, showing different patterns of brain activity in the ADHD-diagnosed and non-ADHD children, also allowed the authors to hypothesize a localized difference in ADHD versus non-ADHD brain function. In their words, as stated in the paper's abstract,

> Findings support the hypothesis of deficient inhibitory control in children with attention-deficit/hyperactivity disorder. Slower inhibitory processing appears to be due to a specific neural deficiency that manifests in the process of the stop signal as attenuated negativity in the N2 latency range (1345).

This conclusion embeds values. One way in which it does so—the values embedded in the stop task itself—will be discussed under "Methodologies," below. Focusing here on language, the thick ethical term "deficient" immediately signals the conclusion's negative value valence. The authors support this value valence by contextualizing their findings. In the paper's introduction, to establish the clinical relevance of their research, they list socially disapproved behaviors exhibited by ADHD-diagnosed children: "Impulsive behaviors typically seen in children with ADHD include impatience, responding before adequate information has been obtained, being easily distracted, and failing to correct inappropriate responses" (Dimoska et al., 2003, 1345). The next sentence states the basic hypothesis their work supports: "Poor inhibitory control has been implicated as a potential core deficit in this disorder, resulting in the observed hyperactivity-impulsivity ADHD symptom pattern" (1345). Two slides in usage subtly introduce value valence. First, the abstract referred to "slow" inhibitory processing; this statement substitutes the value-valenced term "poor." (Faster is *better*.) Second, although they do not equate the commonsense concept of frowned-upon impulsivity and the technical term "inhibitory control," the authors do *correlate* the two terms.[7] By correlating the two—where there is "impulsive behavior" there is "poor inhibitory control"—the value valence of the former attaches to the latter. Such correlations and slides in usage contextualize technical language, and *indirectly embed* values in scientific conclusions.

The standard science-writing tendency to universalize also adds context—hence, context-associated values. Dimoska et al.'s study included 26 children: 13 ADHD-diagnosed and 13 controls. In generalizing their conclusion to all ADHD-diagnosed children, the authors begin to draw on readers' (and their own) associations with environments in which millions of children live and are diagnosed.

The pattern of correlating scientific observations with clinically disvalued traits or behaviors is common in the ADHD science literature. To take one example, such links are frequently made in studies that use structural MRI to examine differences in brain structure between ADHD-diagnosed and non-diagnosed individuals. (Functional MRI, which yields images of the brain "lighting up" because of increased metabolic activity, uses additional technologies to study brain function rather than structure.) Analogously to the stop-task study, the correlation typically indicates the possible clinical significance of the structural differences. For example, Castellanos et al. correlate brain volume differences with the severity of key clinical findings: "Frontal and temporal gray matter, caudate, and cerebellar *volumes* correlated significantly with parent- and clinician-rated *severity measures* within the ADHD sample...(Castellanos et al., 2002, emphasis added, 1740)." Similarly, Pliszka et al. (2006) link clinical behavior and measures of inattentiveness, attention, and inhibition to MRI-studied caudate volumes: "When the left, but not right, *caudate volume* was smaller, the child showed more difficulty in *restless/impulsive behavior* while scores on a *measure of inattentiveness* correlated with *caudate volume* bilaterally...This result is consistent with previous findings of the relationship of smaller left *caudate volume* and *poorer performance on measures of attention and inhibition*", (emphasis added, 1026). Other authors in this subfield associate enlarged hippocampi (Plessen et al., 2006), global and regional thinning of the cortex (Shaw et al., 2006), total cerebral volume (Durston et al., 2004), and brain size and gray matter in the occipital lobe (Sowell et al., 2003) with clinically disvalued traits or "poor" performance on laboratory tests. In each case, the initially neutral finding of structural difference takes on value valence by virtue of its correlation with a clinical problem.

Use of thick ethical terms, subtle assumptions and interpretive shifts, and correlation of data with socially and/or clinically disvalued traits or behaviors is commonplace in the ADHD science literature. These processes embed values in the conclusions of individual articles. But they also build on each other.

More associations can be found, repeated study reinforces the associations, and eventually a network of correlated findings can be drawn on to signal negative valence. The concept "ADHD" itself has negative valence, but after study, so do slower stop task performance, "poor" performance on CPTs, or possession of a specific allele (a "susceptibility gene" that puts individuals "at risk" for ADHD) (Langley et al., 2004). With enough repeated correlation, anatomic differences could also take on value valence. As long as the research keeps finding such correlations, it reinforces existing valences and adds to the store of negative associations. The valencing process proceeds relatively unnoticed and unhindered because the values in question are so widely shared: most agree that faster *is* better when it comes to processing speed; that being easily distracted is bad; and that restless/impulsive behavior is often detrimental or dangerous. But shared values are still values.

Core Methodology/Constitutive Values

The core methodologies of clinical science have a deeper effect on science's conclusions than is often appreciated. For each study, researchers choose methodologies—one or more of the myriad techniques and protocols used in clinical and preclinical (animal) research—with the goals of that particular study in mind. Usually, though, prior research has established that the methods meet key scientific standards for objectivity and reliability. Methods that do not meet these standards, such as poorly constructed survey questions, occasionally appear in the literature, but any biased results these introduce can be dismissed as "bad" science. The more interesting—and more pervasive—cases are those in which methodology is "good" by scientific criteria but nonetheless contributes to the value valence of scientific conclusions. What follows is not an exhaustive list of such cases, but several examples that show the effect.

One way methodology can contribute to the valence of scientific conclusions is by making different evidence available. Elizabeth Anderson compares the methodologies of two groups studying the effects of divorce on women and their children (Anderson, 2004). The method of the "traditionalist" group, which was committed to a two-parent model of family, was to assess objective data, such as post-divorce income levels, at a single time point (a cross-sectional study). The "feminist" group was open to the idea that a variety of family structures could be functional. These researchers supplemented objective data with subjective data, gathered at more than one time (a longitudinal study). Another methodological difference was that the traditionalist researchers analyzed the data in terms of main effects, but the feminist researchers opted to investigate interaction effects. The difference, as Anderson put it, is, "A main effects analysis accepts the average outcome as representative of the group, discounting individual variation. This makes sense if one believes that a single way of life is best for everyone. But for researchers who doubt this, attention to within-groups heterogeneity [for example, by analysis of interaction effects] is imperative..." (17).

The two groups reached different conclusions. The traditionalists found that at the time studied, single-parent families had objective (in the senses of commonly agreed to and unambiguously ascertainable) struggles, such as decreased family income. These researchers concluded that divorce was detrimental to families. The feminists also noted the decreased family income. But their supplementary subjective data, gathered longitudinally, found that many of the women surveyed reported compensating positives, such as more control over the income they did have. Hence, the researchers' conclusions reflected mitigating factors. The feminist researchers' analysis of data in terms of interaction effects as well as main effects showed that outcome varied in interpretable ways among their subjects. In short, each group reached conclusions consonant with their own values. Importantly, this did not result from overt bias in the methodology. Either group's data could have contradicted their expected outcomes: The traditionalists might have found that single-parent families were objectively thriving; the feminist researchers might have found few positives objectively, subjectively, over time, or among subgroups. But the methodology each group employed contributed to the evidence available, hence to the reasonable interpretations of the data. By making available evidence that lets scientists reach a value-valenced conclusion more readily, the methodology contributes to the value valence.

An example from the ADHD literature makes the point clearly. Experts debate whether ADHD is a permanent dysfunction or a developmental delay that "normalizes" over time. Either could result in distinctive neuroanatomy, visible by structural MRI. A cross-sectional MRI study can show structural differences from "controls" at a single time; if the differences are permanent, the specific timing does not matter. But detecting the process of normalization by MRI requires that studies be longitudinal—repeated, in this case, over a period of years. Both types of study have been performed. Based on cross-sectional studies, Mostofsky et al. (2002) and Durston et al. (2004) report, respectively, that ADHD-diagnosed children have a 4% reduction in intracranial volume relative to controls and an 8.3% smaller total cerebral volume. But based on the results of their longitudinal study, Shaw et al. (2007) suggest that most neural structures "catch up" as children mature. Each research group also suggests hypotheses concerning the pathophysiology of ADHD:

"More than one subdivision of the frontal lobes appears to be reduced in volume, suggesting that the clinical picture of ADHD encompasses dysfunctions attributable to anomalous development of both premotor and prefrontal cortices." (Mostofsky et al., 2002, 785)

"The reduction of intracranial volume suggests that the global reduction in brain volume associated with ADHD is related to a relatively early effect." (Durston et al., 2004, 337)

"[Cross-sectional and longitudinal neuroanatomic data sets]...may also guide the future search for factors that delay, rather than derail, cortical development." (Shaw et al., 2007, 19652)

The authors are well aware of the limitations of their methodologies, and they state their hypotheses carefully, not claiming definitive conclusions. Still, Mostofsky et al. and Durston et al., using cross-sectional methodology, lean toward a static view of ADHD's etiology, suggesting permanent dysfunction: they propose "reduced...volume" from "anomalous development" and "global reduction" from a "relatively early effect." Their methodology does not offer evidence about long-term change, and in downplaying the need for such evidence, their hypotheses embed the static view. Shaw et al., however, suggest that there might be "factors that delay, rather than derail, cortical development." By using a method that emphasizes interests in longer-term prognosis or processes, these authors introduce additional evidence, which allows them to support the alternative hypothesis of developmental delay.

As in Anderson's example, all of the research teams use scientifically acceptable methods, but, because they introduce different evidence, the contrasting methodologies encourage contrasting interpretations.[8] But are these interpretations valenced by values? Arguably yes. The static view is consonant with uniform approaches to ADHD, aligning it with categorical views and a sharp focus on individual dysfunction. The developmental view fits less neatly with this model, in that uniform approaches would likely be inappropriate over time, and categorical models would not easily account for gradual change. Earlier chapters detail the many values embedded in these contrasting views: the alignments here continue the valencing process.

Methodology may also valence scientific conclusions via operationalizations that embed values (operationalizations represent immeasurable constructs with measurable data; e.g., IQ tests may represent intelligence). In some operationalizations, the desirable direction of variation in a measured quantity or trait is predetermined. Various intelligence tests have this feature—a *higher* score indicates that the test taker is *smarter*. So does the operationalization of "efficacy" in clinical ADHD drug research. Having *more* symptoms, *more severe* symptoms, or exhibiting symptoms *more often* is considered undesirable; having *fewer* symptoms, *less severe* symptoms, or exhibiting them *less often* is preferred. An "effective" drug therefore *reduces* the number, severity, or frequency of symptoms. When efficacy is operationalized as sitting still (reducing symptoms of hyperactivity) and remaining focused on classroom assignments (reducing symptoms of inattention), the operationalization embeds a positive valuation of children's sitting still and focusing on assignments. If a study's methodology uses a value-valenced operationalization, its conclusions will embed the value valence. In addition, the perceived importance of the chosen endpoints elevates the perceived significance of the research and the findings. Often, in the case of ADHD research, operationalizations embed widely shared social values, such as work and educational standards for achievement, or widely shared medical values, such as concern for an individual's impairment relative to those standards.

Perhaps the most influential way methodology embeds values is via the process of dichotomization that contributes to scientific understanding of a phenomenon.[9] Study designs that seek differences between an affected group and a control group, such as comparing "ADHD" and "normal" or "community control" groups, contribute to the groups' gradually being understood as *more different*—that is, to their dichotomization. The statistical techniques used in such studies are designed to detect differences—even a result of "no significant difference" is (rightly) not interpreted as finding a similarity but as a failure of the hypothesis that the groups differ. As researchers detect differences, they add the differences to the distinctive features attributed to the "ADHD" group. This very typical approach to refining knowledge of ADHD has been repeated in thousands of studies that have investigated hundreds of parameters. Scientists have sought differences in neuroanatomy, genes, neurotransmitters, behavior, school success, driving ability, friendships (etc., etc.). Even when the differences are small, with much overlap between groups—as is empirically the case between ADHD and non-ADHD groups on any given parameter—the accumulation of differences sharpens the distinction between the groups.

Cumulatively, this process dichotomizes "ADHD" from its contrasts. Indirectly, the value valence of "ADHD" also sharpens, because the ascribed features retain the values embedded by other means (investigative trends, background assumptions, operationalizations, thick ethical terms, and so forth), and the dichotomization locates them in one group and not the other—that is, it becomes clearer to whom the normative judgments attached to differences apply. The sharpening and clarification of differences also indirectly reinforces the idea that the features are accurately described—and the relevant values are accurately ascribed. The interest in finding differences, making distinctions, and developing categories—the impetus that encourages dichotomization—is itself also value valenced.[10] This is difficult to see, as it is such a pervasive pattern in Western thinking and practice (even toddlers sort their blocks!), but considering the contrast with non-dichotomizing world views, such as Buddhist perspectives, can highlight the valence.

Statistical analysis focusing on group averages rather than intragroup variation sharpens dichotomization. Often, researchers have no choice—if funding dictates a small sample size, for example, intragroup analyses may not be possible. Nevertheless, the group average sometimes homogenizes significant intragroup differences. For example, extremes of variation or clusters within the average may suggest (or require) explanations that the average alone does not. Even modest variation may be relevant to a problem—especially a clinical problem, where individuals matter. This means that even research that takes steps to address variation may be critiqued as inadequately individualized. For example, the major Multimodal Treatment Study of Children With Attention-Deficit/Hyperactivity Disorder (MTA) considered four different forms of intervention for ADHD: a careful titration of medication ("medical management"), behavioral management, both medical and behavioral management ("combined treatment"), and community care, which in practice consisted of medication less carefully titrated than that in the medical management group. In many of the papers based on this protocol, the research team expresses its conclusions as group averages, or subdivides the results according to a limited number of factors. For example, "'normalization' rates" 14 months after the beginning of the study are stated for all children in each care group (56%, 34%, 68%, and 25%, respectively) and also are subdivided according to comorbid internalizing disorders, externalizing disorders, or both (Jensen et al., 2005, 1631). Yet the team also takes care to consider variables that might affect individual outcomes. They found, for example, that children who had symptoms of anxiety in addition to their ADHD fared better with behavior therapy than with community care, and that families' acceptance of treatment and attendance at sessions affected outcomes (Jensen et al., 2007; MTA Cooperative Group, 1999). But these analyses are still averages within averages. Regarding research on intervention, some investigators think that studying individual responses is crucial, given individual variation in relevant traits, behaviors, and reactions to treatment; the individual's location in a family and social system; and the effects on the individual and the system of small changes in behavior. "Clearly," writes one such researcher, "pitting one treatment against another perpetuates the notion that one size fits all, and adds little to our knowledge of children and development"

(Heriot, Evans, & Foster, 2007, 129). There are positive reasons for *not* undertaking individual-centered analyses—individual variation can hide important information by missing a crucial trend in a sea of detail. In any case, such methods are not representative of current scientific practice. Because most methodologies generalize and dichotomize, individual members of a group begin to be perceived—by scientists, and by the clinicians and public to whom scientific findings are disseminated—as relevantly similar to one another.

Although researchers and clinicians are well aware that generalizations based on averages do not necessarily apply to any specific individual, generalizations are nevertheless a common feature of scientific and clinical discourse. For example, in an article discussing the psychosocial treatments to be used in the MTA the authors write, "Furthermore, despite the early prevailing view that ADHD was a time-limited disorder of prepuberty, prospective studies on psychiatric clinic samples have revealed ADHD to be a chronic disorder in a substantial majority of children who have the diagnosis, with antisocial outcomes, substance abuse, and continued attentional, family, interpersonal, and occupational difficulties persisting into adolescence and adulthood" (Wells et al., 2000, 484). Again, the MTA authors temper their generalizations with the phrases "psychiatric clinical samples" and "a substantial majority"—reminders to readers that not all ADHD-diagnosed children will experience the outcomes they list. Yet the paragraph from which the sentence is taken concerns the general features of the disorder, raising the expectation that the features reported describe the universe of ADHD-diagnosed people. Further, although the authors mention the source of the sample they discuss, they do not explain the potential difference between a psychiatric clinical sample, which would be expected to consist of relatively severe cases, and a community sample. This combination (the intent to review general features and the unexplained limitation of the sample) implies that the findings of the psychiatric clinical sample pertain to all ADHD-diagnosed individuals: ADHD risks seem worse, for all patients, after reading that ADHD is (in a substantial majority of a psychiatric clinic sample) associated with various undesirable outcomes. Notably, generalizations get picked up in clinical practice as well. For example, clinical practice guidelines produced by the American Academy of Pediatrics (AAP) and the American Academy of Child and Adolescent Psychiatry (AACAP) make generalized recommendations based on data that itself typically reports generalizations (AACAP, 2002; AAP, 2001; Pliszka et al., 2007).[11]

The result of the generalizing is a form of stereotyping, in which members of the ADHD group are typed according to the diagnostic criteria used to select them, according to the average results of individual studies, and according to the values embedded in the research. The MTA team and authors of guidelines *know* that average values do not necessarily reflect an individual's traits or outcomes, yet the discourse they practice, reiterated by others, establishes a default for quick judgments: the default becomes the averages expressed.

At least since 1980, ADHD research has embedded values in its operationalizations, methodologies, hypotheses, and conclusions. The result has been the decades-long accretion of negative values to the standard view of ADHD.[12] By studying DSM-modeled ADHD to the near exclusion of other possibilities, the sciences have not stood apart from the multiple values associated with social interests in ADHD or even taken available steps to decrease or diffuse the influence of values. The quotes that opened the chapter, representative of similar thousands, show the negative valence stemming from social, medical, and scientific influences: "Susceptibility" genes are undesirable, as is ADHD's interference with potential and achievement.[13] The term "barriers" makes sense only if the parents *should* endorse the espoused view of ADHD. "No support" is offered according to the criteria used in the study, but the blanket statement suggests a strong assumption that those criteria can be universalized. Finally, "cost-effectiveness" embeds multiple assumptions about cost and efficacy—and regard for cost-effectiveness as a goal.

Yet the sciences have potential to change these patterns and their influence. I will argue in Chapter 6 that seeking value freedom is not the means to do this; the clinical sciences in general cannot reach the ideal of pure scientific objectivity. But this "failure" by itself is not a problem; instead, it is the particular values that imbue ADHD science that are undesirable, given that they reinforce intolerance (*see* Chapter 5). To counter this, scientists might study differently conceived groups, diffusing or redistributing values in the process. Or they might explore more aspects of ADHD, or more often focus on variation within ADHD-diagnosed groups, with similar results. The alternatives would embed values as well, but those values would likely differ from those associated with today's ADHD, and the existence of alternatives might loosen the present pattern.

The Feedback Loop

I close this chapter with a central point. Earlier chapters showed that scientific views affect other social institutions and practices, including the practices of medicine and education. This chapter clarifies that the influence is mutual: Needs and interests in medical, educational, and other social venues deeply affect the practice and conclusions of science. The result is a positive feedback loop (*see* Fig. 4.1) that, to date, has worked to strengthen the negative valence ascribed to ADHD. As we will see in Chapter 5, the negative views, certified by science, are directed to ADHD-diagnosable people as well: The feedback loop reinforces intolerance.

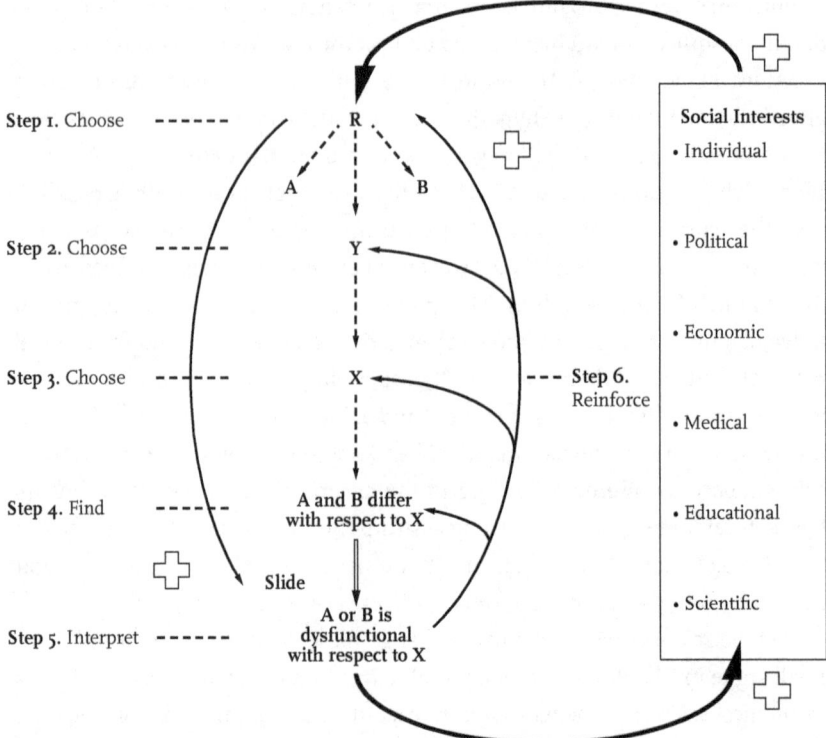

FIGURE 4.1 A positive feedback loop embeds values in scientific constructs, operationalizations, interpretations, and conclusions. The pattern applies, to varying degrees, to all successful clinical sciences, given the values embedded in topics of clinical interest. Here the first step is choosing to study topic R, ADHD, according to the common protocol of dividing the groups studied into affected and non-affected groups A and B (e.g., ADHD and non-ADHD). Protocols other than the A/B division also embed values; the figure simplifies for purposes of illustration.). The division adds values associated with dichotomization to values that mark R as a phenomenon of interest. More specific choices of what to study—such as topic Y (e.g., attention) and the operationalization X (e.g., continuous performance tests)—also embed values. Thus, even at the point that a "difference" is found between A and B, the observed difference is only relatively value-free, having been arrived at through several value-valenced choices. The slide from "difference" to "dysfunction," the latter a thick ethical term, intensifies the value valence. The positive result of the study reinforces the original choice to study R, Y, and X, strengthening the feedback loop. Meanwhile, social interests intensify the reinforcement, thousands of repetitions of the feedback loop tighten the enmeshment of fact and value, and the enmeshments and positive results of the science reinforce the social interests. (A version of this figure appeared as Figure 2, p. 27, in Hawthorne, S. (2010), Embedding Values: How Science and Society Jointly Valence a Concept—the Case of ADHD," *Studies in the History and Philosophy of Biology and the Biomedical Sciences* 41:21–31.)

REFERENCES

American Academy of Child and Adolescent Psychiatry (2002). AACAP Official Action: Practice parameter for the use of stimulant medications in the treatment of children, adolescents, and adults. *Journal of the American Academy of Child and Adolescent Psychiatry*, 41(Suppl 2), 26S–49S.

American Academy of Pediatrics, Committee on Quality Improvement, Subcommittee on Attention-Deficit/Hyperactivity Disorder (2001). Clinical practice guideline: treatment of the school-aged child with attention-deficit/hyperactivity disorder. *Pediatrics*, 108(4), 1033–1044.

American Psychiatric Association (2000). *Diagnostic and Statistical Manual of Mental Disorders* (4, Text Revision ed.). Arlington, VA: American Psychiatric Association.

American Psychiatric Association (2013). *Diagnostic and Statistical Manual of Mental Disorders: DSM-5* (5th ed.). Washington, DC: American Psychiatric Association.

Anderson, E. (2004). Uses of value judgments in science: a general argument, with lessons from a case study of feminist research on divorce. *Hypatia*, 19(1), 1–24.

Barry, T. D., Lyman, R. D., & Klinger, L. G. (2002). Academic underachievement and attention-deficit/hyperactivity disorder: the negative impact of symptom severity on school performance. *Journal of School Psychology*, 40(3), 259–283.

Biederman, J., & Faraone, S. V. (2006). The Effects of Attention-Deficit/Hyperactivity Disorder on Employment and Household Income. *Medscape General Medicine*, 8(3), 12. Retrieved September 7, 2007, from http://www.medscape.com/viewarticle/536264

Bussing, R., Gary, F. A., Mills, T. L., & Garvan, C. W. (2003). Parental explanatory models of ADHD: Gender and cultural variations. *Social Psychiatry and Psychiatric Epidemiology*, 38, 563–575.

Castellanos, F. X., Lee, P. P., Sharp, W., Jeffries, N. O., Greenstein, D. K., Clasen, L. S., et al. (2002). Developmental trajectories of brain volume abnormalities in children and adolescents with attention-deficit/hyperactivity disorder. *JAMA*, 288(14), 1740–1748.

Chesapeake Institute (1993). *Executive Summaries of Research Syntheses and Promising Practices on the Education of Children with Attention Deficit Disorder*. Washington, D.C.: Chesapeake Institute.

Dimoska, A., Johnstone, S. J., Barry, R. J., & Clarke, A. R. (2003). Inhibitory motor control in children with attention-deficit/hyperactivity disorder: event-related potentials in the stop-signal paradigm. *Biological Psychiatry*, 54, 1345–1354.

DuPaul, G. (2007). School-based interventions for students with attention deficit hyperactivity disorder: current status and future directions. *School Psychology Review*, 36(2), 183–194.

Durston, S., Pol, H. E. H., Schnack, H. G., Buitelaar, J. K., Steenhuis, M. P., Minderaa, R. B., et al. (2004). Magnetic resonance imaging of boys with attention-deficit/hyperactivity disorder and their unaffected siblings. *Journal of the American Academy of Child and Adolescent Psychiatry*, 43(3), 332–340.

Evans, S. W. (2005). Introduction to special issue on school-based treatment of children and adolescents with ADHD. *Journal of Attention Disorders, 9*(1), 245–247.

Faraone, S. V., Doyle, A. E., Mick, E., & Biederman, J. (2001). Meta-analysis of the association between the 7-repeat allele of the dopamine D(4) receptor gene and attention deficit hyperactivity disorder. *Am J Psychiatry, 158*(7), 1052–1057.

Fries, J. F., & Krishnan, E. (2004). Equipoise, design bias, and randomized controlled trials: the elusive ethics of new drug development. *Arthritis Res Ther, 6*(3), R250–R255.

Furman, L. M. (2008). Attention-deficit hyperactivity disorder (ADHD): does new research support old concepts? *J Child Neurol, 23*(7), 775–784.

Gannett, L. (2001). Racism and human genome diversity research: the ethical limits of 'population thinking'. *Philosophy of Science, 68*(Supplement), S479–S492.

Hechtman, L., Abikoff, H. B., Klein, R. G., Weiss, G., Respitz, C., Kouri, J., et al. (2004). Academic achievement and emotional status of children with ADHD treated with long-term methylphenidate and multimodal psychosocial treatment. *Journal of the American Academy of Child and Adolescent Psychiatry, 43*(7), 812–819.

Heriot, S. A., Evans, I. M., & Foster, T. M. (2007). Critical influences affecting response to various treatments in young children with ADHD: a case series. *Child: care, health and development, 34*(1), 121–133.

Jensen, P. S., Arnold, L. E., Swanson, J. M., Vitiello, B., Abikoff, H. B., Greenhill, L. L., et al. (2007). 3-year follow-up of the NIMH MTA study. *Journal of the American Academy of Child and Adolescent Psychiatry, 46*(8), 989–1002.

Jensen, P. S., Garcia, J. A., Glied, S., Crowe, M., Foster, M., Schlander, M., et al. (2005). Cost-effectiveness of ADHD treatments: Findings from the Multimodal Treatment Study of Children with ADHD. *American Journal of Psychiatry, 162*(9), 1628–1636.

Kelly, R. E., Cohen, L. J., Semple, R. J., Bodenheimer, A., Neustadter, E., Barenboim, A., et al. (2006). Relationship between drug company funding and outcomes of clinical psychiatric research. *Psychological Medicine, 36*, 1647–1656.

Krimsky, S. (2003). *Science in the Private Interest: Has the Lure of Corporate Profit Corrupted Biomedical Research?* Lanham, MD: Rowman & Littlefield.

Kuhn, T. S. (1996 [1962]). *The Structure of Scientific Revolutions* (3 ed.). Chicago: University of Chicago Press.

Langley, K., Marshall, L., van den Bree, M., Thomas, H., Owen, M., O'Donovan, M., et al. (2004). Association of the dopamine D4 receptor gene 7-repeat allele with neuropsychological test performance of children with ADHD. *American Journal of Psychiatry, 161*(1), 133–138.

Lemmens, T. (2004). Leopards in the Temple: Restoring Scientific Integrity to the Commercialized Research Scene. *Journal of Law, Medicine, and Ethics, 32*(4), 641–657.

Lexchin, J., Bero, L. A., Djulbegovic, B., & Clark, O. (2003). Pharmaceutical industry sponsorship and research outcome and quality: systematic review. *British Medical Journal, 326*, 1167–1170.

Longino, H. E. (1990). *Science as Social Knowledge: Values and Objectivity in Scientific Inquiry.* Princeton, NJ: Princeton University Press.

Mayes, R., Bagwell, C., & Erkulwater, J. (2009). *Medicating Children: ADHD and Pediatric Mental Health*. Cambridge, MA: Harvard University Press.

Melander, H., Ahlqvist-Rastad, J., Meijer, G., & Beermann, B. (2004). Evidence b(i)ased medicine—selective reporting from studies sponsored by pharmaceutical industry: review of studies in new drug applications. *British Medical Journal, 326*, 1171–1173.

Mostofsky, S. H., Cooper, K. L., Kates, W. R., Denckla, M. B., & Kaufmann, W. E. (2002). Smaller prefrontal and premotor volumes in boys with attention deficit/hyperactivity disorder. *Biological Psychiatry, 52*, 785–794.

MTA Cooperative Group (1999). Moderators and mediators of treatment response for children with attention-deficit/hyperactivity disorder: The multimodal treatment study of children with attention-deficit/hyperactivity disorder. *Archives of General Psychiatry, 56*, 1088–1096.

Oades, R. D. (2007). The role of the serotonin system in ADHD: treatment implications. *Expert Review of Neurotherapeutics, 7*(10), 1357–1374.

Pelham, W. E., & Fabiano, G. A. (2008). Evidence-based psychosocial treatments for attention-deficit/hyperactivity disorder. *Journal of Clinical Child and Adolescent Psychology, 37*(1), 184–214.

Peppercorn, J., Blood, E., Winer, E., & Partridge, A. (2007). Association between pharmaceutical involvement and outcomes in breast cancer clinical trials. *Cancer, 109*(7), 1239–1246

Plessen, K. J., Bansal, R., Zhu, H., Whiteman, R., Amat, J., Quackenbush, G. A., et al. (2006). Hippocampus and amygdala morphology in attention-deficit/hyperactivity disorder. *Arch Gen Psychiatry, 63*(7), 795–807.

Pliszka, S., Bernet, W., Bukstein, O., Walter, H. J., Arnold, V., Beitchman, J., et al. (2007). Practice parameter for the assessment and treatment of children and adolescents with attention-deficit/hyperactivity disorder *Journal of the American Academy of Child and Adolescent Psychiatry, 46*(7), 894–921.

Pliszka, S. R., Lancaster, J., Liotti, M., & Semrud-Clikeman, M. (2006). Volumetric MRI differences in treatment-naive vs chronically treated children with ADHD. *Neurology, 67*(6), 1023–1027.

Putnam, H. (2002). *The Collapse of the Fact/Value Dichotomy and Other Essays*. Cambridge, MA: Harvard University Press.

Rubia, K. (2005). RED: ADHD under the "micro-scope" of the rat model. *Behavioral and Brain Sciences, 28*(3), 439–440.

Sagvolden, T., Aase, H., Johansen, E. B., & Russell, V. A. (2005). A dynamic developmental theory of attention-deficit/hyperactivity disorder (ADHD) predominantly hyperactive/impulsive and combined subtypes. *Behavioral and Brain Sciences, 28*(3), 397–468.

Shaw, P., Eckstrand, K., Sharp, W., Blumenthal, J., Lerch, J. P., Greenstein, D., et al. (2007). Attention-deficit/hyperactivity disorder is characterized by a delay in cortical maturation. *Proceedings of the National Academy of Science, 104*(49), 19,649–19,654.

Shaw, P., Lerch, J., Greenstein, D., Sharp, W. S., Clasen, L., Evans, A., et al. (2006). Longitudinal Mapping of Cortical Thickness and Clinical Outcome in Children and Adolescents With Attention-Deficit/Hyperactivity Disorder. *Arch Gen Psychiatry, 63*(5), 540–549.

Sowell, E. R., Thompson, P. M., Welcome, S. E., Henkenius, A. L., Toga, A. W., & Peterson, B. S. (2003). Cortical abnormalities in children and adolescents with attention-deficit hyperactivity disorder. *The Lancet, 362*(9397), 1699–1707.

Tripp, G., & Wickens, J. R. (2009). Neurobiology of ADHD. *Neuropharmacology, 57*(7–8), 579–589.

Wells, K. C., Pelham, W. E., Kotkin, R. A., Hoza, B., Abikoff, H. B., Abramowitz, A., et al. (2000). Psychosocial treatment strategies in the MTA study: Rationale, methods, and critical issues in design and implementation. *Journal of Abnormal Child Psychology, 28*(6), 483–505.

Wilens, T. E. (2008). Effects of methylphenidate on the catecholaminergic system in attention-deficit/hyperactivity disorder. *J Clin Psychopharmacol, 28*(3 Suppl 2), S46–S53.

NOTES

1. *See* Chapter 1 for details.
2. I use the term "value valence" rather than "value laden" because the latter term has two connotations I want to resist: the first is that the values in question are bad values—in clinical science the values in question are often widely agreed to. The second is that sciences' being affected by values is bad. This is sometimes the case, but because the effects are inevitable, care is needed to discover when and why it is problematic, rather than implying that it always is so.
3. *See* Chapter 2, which explored the current research and future goals of the sciences in isolation from medicine and wider society, and Chapters 1 and 3, which examined medical and social aspects of ADHD, respectively.
4. *See* Chapter 2 for a discussion of what counts as evidence in the sciences of ADHD.
5. To assess the focus of the ADHD intervention literature, I searched the ERIC, PsychINFO, and Medline databases for journal articles appearing in the years 2001 through 2005 that had "ADHD" or "attention-deficit/hyperactivity disorder" in the title. I then imported the results from each search into the bibliographic program EndNote and eliminated duplicate references. This left a set of 2,749 articles that had appeared in 712 journals. I used the program JMP to count the number of articles per journal. I searched the 1,300 articles (47% of the total) from those journals that published more than 2 articles matching the search criteria by keywords chosen to count articles related to academic/educational, behavioral, or pharmacological interventions.
6. The second, third, and fourth factors were: varying ADD criteria, varied and unaccounted-for comorbidities, and underrepresentation of girls.

7. Technically, "inhibitory control" refers to a construct for which the underlying neural structures are somewhat localizable by EEG. Inhibitory control is the process that can, given enough time after a stimulus, interrupt the "response process" that reacts to the same or a different stimulus.
8. Because cross-sectional methods do not convey a developmental picture, it is *possible* to frankly bias one's conclusions by only considering cross-sectional data. This possibility is very clearly understood among scientists, and Mostofsky et al. and Durston et al. take care to distance themselves from such bias.
9. *See* Chapters 1 and 2 for reasons dichotomization is methodologically common; *see* Chapter 5 for effect of this emphasis on ADHD-diagnosable people.
10. Once again, we also see that the concept of "difference" is only relatively value-free.
11. The AAP's guideline and the AACAP's 2007 practice parameter address treatment of school-aged children with ADHD; AACAP's 2002 practice parameter concerns use of stimulant medications more generally, but is directed primarily at ADHD therapy. (American Academy of Child and Adolescent Psychiatry, 2002; American Academy of Pediatrics, 2001; Pliszka et al., 2007)
12. The pattern has held despite the concern of some scientists that the DSM models have been and are inadequate (*see* Chapters 1 and 2).
13. The quote from Barry, Lyman et al. (2002) dichotomizes less than the others, given that it suggests that children with a subthreshold level of ADHD-associated symptoms might also benefit from educational interventions. This is, in my view, less a counterexample to my claim that the ADHD sciences dichotomize than an illustration that the view among psychologists, including school psychologists, is less dichotomized than that among psychiatrists. *See* Chapter 5 for additional discussion of this point.

5   ACCIDENTAL INTOLERANCE

How does the current understanding of ADHD affect diagnosable people? According to the predominant view, current understanding and practice have reduced the stigma associated with ADHD-type traits and behaviors and allow affected people struggling in school or at work to get needed help. The idea is that scientific/medical understanding of mental disorder removes moral or moralistic framing: ADHD-diagnosable children are no longer considered "naughty" or their parents as "poor" or "neglectful"; diagnosable adults are not "underachievers." Rather, those affected simply have a biological constitution that predisposes them to certain dysfunctional traits and behaviors, and the response should be clinical care. The rapid uptake of diagnosis and treatment over the past 20 years corroborates the welcome that clinicians, ADHD-diagnosable people, and parents have given to this understanding.

The present situation can be read differently, however. As previous chapters have argued, the current understanding of ADHD retains negative values. Rather than removing the value-valenced attitudes, the joint influences of science and society have reinforced the negative associations with ADHD. This chapter suggests that the consistent reinforcement has an unintended effect—it feeds intolerance of ADHD-associated traits and behaviors and naturalizes disvaluing those traits and behaviors (and the people who exhibit them) by institutionalizing ways to detect them. If this is the case, the uptake of the diagnosis is not pure welcome, but at least in part acquiescence to institutionalized intolerance. The "intolerance" is not the old stigma—it is a biologized and medicalized disvaluation, rather than an overtly moral one. Yet continued negative perceptions of ADHD, and the ways those perceptions contribute to limiting ADHD-diagnosable people's options, constitute a new form of intolerance.

Few purposefully cultivate such attitudes,[1] which are instead an accidental byproduct of current and past practice. Non-majority views also complicate the picture. For example, ADHD skeptics who doubt the "reality" of ADHD, those opposed to pharmacotherapy, and sometimes even those who more moderately doubt aspects or degrees of current concepts and practices, also pressure ADHD-diagnosed people—but toward rejection of diagnosis and treatment, rather than uptake. Such alternative perspectives may be a prominent part of any given individual's experience and choices. But these crosscutting views are not institutionalized in education, medicine, or other aspects of society. For this reason, although this chapter discusses non-majority views (*see* "The Drug Wars and Skeptics' Intolerance," below), the focus is on how the institutionalized view affects ADHD-diagnosable people's lives.

Perspectives on ADHD

We all live in cultures constituted by concepts, institutions, and practices; our lives are shaped by this complex mix. Looking again at the aspects of culture that have grown up around ADHD—especially at the values embedded in our concepts, institutions, and practices—helps us understand effects on ADHD-diagnosable people. The perspectives and practices adopted by the majority present some options and close off others, both in terms of practical choices and in terms of self-concept. (Again, later sections will consider minority views and their effects.)

We have already seen that the predominant understanding of ADHD is highly normative. For many years, evaluative language and concepts have colored the professional literatures that instituted and refined the category, embedding goals implicitly or explicitly valued goals. Medical literature of the 1970s, when the ADHD precursors were termed "hyperkinesis" or "minimal brain dysfunction," described the affected children using terms such as "disobedient," "moody," "irritable," "clumsy," "inattentive," or "driven" (in the sense of lack of control or agency; *see* Table 5.1) (Aronson, 1971; Eisenberg, 1972; Kenny et al., 1971; Schulte, 1971; Towbin, 1971; Wikler, Dixon, & Parker, 1970). Similarly, the 1970s education literature used terms such as "acting out," "ill-mannered," and "failure-prone" (Broudy, 1976; Freeman, 1976; Grinspoon & Singer, 1973; Hackett, 1975; Krauch, 1971; Miller, 1973; Renstrom, 1976; Robin & Bosco, 1976; Stewart, 1976). Each of these terms expresses a judgment of the child, mixing the child's behavior with the reaction of an annoyed or concerned adult.

The 2000-era professional literature has become more circumspect. Presumably, most scientists, clinicians, and educators would see themselves

Table 5.1 Adjectives Used to Describe Children Characterized as Having Minimal Brain Dysfunction, Hyperkinetic Impulse Disorder, or ADHD.

1970s, education literature

Exceptional
Dead-end
Acting-out
Ill-mannered
Strange
Uncoordinated
Intelligent
Mercurial
Impatient
Jet propelled
Impossible
Inattentive
Failure-prone
Hyperactive
Problem
Bad
Disordered
Educationally handicapped
Holy terror
Unmanageable
Juvenile delinquent
Disturbed
Restless
Angry
Psychologically or organically sick, deviant, or deficient
Zombie (when taking Ritalin)

1970s, medical literature

Exceptional
Disobedient
Moody, irritable [as baby]
Driven [not free to behave]

(continued)

Table 5.1. (Continued)

Organically rejected; unready and fragile; expressed through a physiologically unprepared, unrelaxed birth canal…pistoned down the birth canal and separated…[when premature]
  Minimal brain damaged
  Clumsy
  Inattentive
  Hyperactive
  Less satiable [...become(s) stimulus-hungry more quickly]
  Physiologically underaroused
  Happy hyperactive

*2000s, education literature**

Fidgety
Loud
Aggressive
Underachiever
Inattentive
Unalienable to adult control

*2000s, medical literature**

Regarding the child:
  Unmedicated or medicated
  ADHD [vs. healthy controls]
Regarding a trait, mechanism, behavior:
  Dysfunctional
  Deficient
  Poor (performance, inhibitory control, etc.)
  Impulsive
  Inattentive

*Traits in this literature typically expressed as something the child "has" or "is characterized by" or that is "in" the child, rather than something the child *is*. Alternatively, adjectives are used to describe the behavior or a mechanism rather than the child.

as assessing children (or adults) rather than judging them, with the overall goal of helping a student or patient. Yet the arguments of previous chapters suggest that judgments like those seen in the 1970s have been tempered but not dispelled. In the education literature, adjectives generally describe something the child "has," or "is characterized by," rather than something s/he "is" (Alban-Metcalfe, Cheng-Lai, & Ma, 2002; Barry, Lyman, & Klinger, 2002; Brand, Dunn, & Greb, 2002; Davison, 2001; Flood & Wilder, 2002; Gresham, Lane, & Lambros, 2000; Purdie, Hattie, & Carroll, 2002; Schirduan, Case, & Faryniarz, 2002; Stinnett, Crawford, Gillespie, Cruce, & Langford, 2001; Xu, Reid, & Steckelberg, 2002). Despite this deflection, though, the normative judgment is clear in terms such as "loud," "aggressive," or "underachiever" (one group [Gresham et al., 2000] used the term "fledgling psychopaths," but such overtly negative terminology is likely frowned on). Authors of the scientific and medical literature generally highlight harm caused to the child by his or her biological dysfunction, and their normative judgments appear more circumspect (Baird, Stevenson, & Williams, 2000; Bastiaansen, Koot, Ferdinand, & Verhulst, 2004; Brewis, 2002; Bussing, Gary, Mills, & Garvan, 2003; Castellanos, et al., 2002; Christakis, Zimmerman, DiGiuseppe, & McCarty, 2004; Ding et al., 2002; Durston et al., 2004; Madras, Miller, & Fischman, 2002; MTA Cooperative Group, 2004a; MTA Cooperative Group, 2004b; Solanto, Arnsten, & Castellanos, 2001; Steger et al., 2000; Swanson et al., 2000; Teicher et al., 2000). They typically refer to children by diagnosis ("ADHD children") or as "subjects" or "patients." Yet the normative judgment remains in effect. In part, value judgments are simply packed into the diagnostic criteria for ADHD, in which children's failures to live up to adult expectations are prominent.[2] More subtly, throughout the research literature, authors describe ADHD children's traits or behaviors in terms such as "deficiencies," "inadequacies," or "excesses" relative to desired norms. Such redescriptions make two switches in emphasis. First, they mute the overtly judgmental terminology of earlier years. Second, the description is generally not of the *child* but of his or her traits or behaviors. However, as we saw in Chapter 4, authors explicitly link such descriptions of their findings to clinically relevant ratings or correlates[3], which are clinically relevant *because* they have value valence (e.g., Dimoska et al. [2003] link "poor inhibitory control" to disvalued "impulsive behavior"). This ensures that normative judgments remain embedded in the terminology—and in the conclusions of the science, as Chapter 4 argued—despite their subtler expression.

Even in the clinical literature, though, the expression of normative judgments is not always particularly subtle. A 1997 book uses the terms automatic, thoughtless, unintentional, ill considered, random, and impulsive to describe the behavior of ADHD-diagnosed children (Barkley, 1997, 248). Barkley also "predicts that those with ADHD will be found to be delayed in the stages of moral development" (249). More recently, Jensen et al. (2005) exemplified the pattern, explaining that "...difficulties experienced by children with ADHD may continue or even increase into adulthood, resulting in possible justice system contacts and substance abuse troubles, as well as effects on ultimate rates of child abuse, crime, adult mental illness, and accidents with severe injuries" (1628). Similarly, questions in the "Adult ADHD Self-Report Scale" place high value on the virtues of persistence, detail orientation, and focused attention, with implied negative judgment of the converses[4] : "How often do you have trouble wrapping up the final details of a project, once the challenging parts have been done?" "How often do you have difficulty keeping your attention when you are doing boring or repetitive work?"

Norms engaged by the diagnostic categories may also be gendered. Some researchers suggest that presentation, course, and treatment varies by sex (Gaub & Carlson, 1997; Graetz, Sawyer, & Baghurst, 2005; Greene et al., 2001; Hinshaw, Carte, Fan, Jassy, & Owens, 2007; Levy, Hay, Bennett, & McStephen, 2005; Newcorn et al., 2001; Ohan & Johnston, 2005; Quinn, 2005; Zalecki & Hinshaw, 2004), and others, that perceptions of parents, teachers, peers, and others do so as well (Bussing, Gary, Mills, & Garvan, 2003; Chen, Seipp, & Johnston, 2008; Quinn & Wigal, 2004; Singh, 2003; Thurber, Heller, & Hinshaw, 2002). Consider the following quotes:

> "Compared with boys, girls are more likely to be inattentive without being excessively hyperactive or impulsive, and hyperactivity in females is more likely to manifest as hypertalkativeness or emotional reactivity than excessive motor activity." (Clarke, Barry, McCarthy, Selikowitz, & Johnstone, 2007, 2701)

> "There are also differences in the profiles of comorbidities, with girls more likely to have comorbid internalizing disorders, and boys more likely to have comorbid externalizing disorders. AD/HD in girls is also more likely to lead to substance abuse disorders and sexual acting out in adolescence." (Clarke et al., 2007, 2701)

> "Women with ADHD tend to have higher rates of adolescent pregnancy and substance abuse than other women, and are more likely than other mothers to provide inattentive, inconsistent, or impulsive caregiving... They may create a toxic or stressful environment for their vulnerable offspring." (Arnold, 1996, 562)

Scientists debate whether the generalizations stated in these quotes are even correct (Derks, Hudziak, & Boomsma, 2007; Novik et al., 2006). More importantly for the present point, the stated patterns of ADHD symptomatology mirror gender stereotypes. The girls are day-dream-y, hypertalkative, and emotionally reactive, with internalizing disorders (such as depression), substance abuse, and "sexual acting out." Diagnosable boys, in contrast, are said to fit a "boys will be boys" hyperactive, impulsive, "externalizing" overgeneralization. That stereotyped boy is also white. Black boys are more likely to be categorized, for the purpose of special education, as "emotionally disturbed" (i.e., aggressive)—again, the categories align with subdivisions and kinds that do not stray too far from common, and pernicious, stereotypes (see Chapter 3).

The professional literature reaches a wide audience. But the pharmaceutical industry also plays a role in publicizing—and often hyping—the messages of scientists, clinicians, and educators about ADHD and other mental illnesses (Angell, 2004; Diller, 2005; Elliott, 2000). Drug company "education" of physicians about the vicissitudes of ADHD-like disorders dates to the 1960s (Cohn, 1971). From these quarters, messages about ADHD can wax hyperbolic—and divisive. For example, a recent drug company-sponsored digital monograph once available for continuing medical education credits for U.S. physicians (Anonymous, 2005a), quotes prominent psychopharmacologist Joseph Biederman as saying, "The evidence that ADHD is an extraordinarily morbid condition is overwhelming...[it is an] enormously morbid, costly, and potentially devastating condition...untreated ADHD carries a very ominous prognosis'" (11–12).

Since the early 1990s, drug companies have also promoted products directly to consumers. ADHD advertisements emphasize both the seriousness of the problem and the benefits of medication. For example, one widely valued skill is the ability to fit into social situations, and ADHD-diagnosed children may lack the kinds of behavioral control typically expected. Picking up on this, McNeil Pharmaceuticals' consumer-oriented DVD about the company's ADHD drug Concerta shows a young person, apparently a Concerta user, saying, "I am much more under control, and [friends] want to be around me. I'm a much nicer person to be around" (McNeil Consumer & Specialty Pharmaceuticals, 2003).

Drug companies also sponsor research designed to get out an urgent normative message. In the United States, self-esteem, quality of life, and net worth are often closely linked. Shire, manufacturer of the ADHD drug Adderall XR, which it promotes for adults, sponsored a "large-scale survey" called "Capturing America's Attention." The survey results were touted in at least two rounds of press releases (Anonymous, 2004); (Anonymous, 2005b), presented at the annual meeting of the American Psychiatric Association, and finally published in 2006 (Biederman & Faraone, 2006). The take-home message of the paper is that adult ADHD costs $67 billion to $116 billion in lost workforce productivity annually: $8,900 to $15,400 per ADHD-diagnosed adult per year. In one of the press releases, the study's spokesperson (Biederman), said that "'ADHD...may be one of the costliest medical conditions in the United States...Evaluating, diagnosing, and treating this condition may not only improve the quality of life, but may save adults with ADHD billions of dollars every year'" (Anonymous, 2005b, unpaginated).

But to return to messages of science, the negative valence attributed to ADHD arises in part because ADHD-typical cognitive and behavioral traits are conceived as "deficits," "deficiencies," or "reductions" relative to a norm—in other words, these ADHD-associated traits are undesirable. Perhaps more influentially, scientists have also observed many negatively perceived, long-term correlates of ADHD diagnosis. These include higher risk of automobile accident and injury (Barkley, Murphy, & Kwasnik, 1996; DiScala, Lescohier, Barthel, & Li, 1998; Leibson, Katusic, Barbaresi, Ransom, & O'Brien, 2001; Woodward, Fergusson, & Horwood, 2000), delinquency or criminality (Molina et al., 2007; Sourander et al., 2006), school failure (Hechtman et al., 2004; Yang, Chung, Chen, & Chen, 2004), reduced income (Biederman & Faraone, 2006), impaired social relations (Abikoff et al., 2004; Ohan & Johnston, 2007), substance abuse (Molina et al., 2007; Wilens, Faraone, Biederman, & Gunawardene, 2003), and high medical costs (Birnbaum et al., 2005; Leibson et al., 2001). Many of these correlates are disvalued by nearly everyone, and most people would also judge that they harm the affected individual as well as wider society. Yet these are statistical associations—any given correlate may or may not apply to a particular individual. Misunderstood as accurate descriptions of individuals—as they often are—such generalizations (1) misrepresent a significant percentage of ADHD-diagnosable people and (2) contribute to a negatively valenced stereotype.

With negative views of ADHD prominent in the professional literatures, and reaching from there to popular media, it is no surprise that some recent studies suggest that ADHD-diagnosed individuals are portrayed and perceived negatively. Danforth and Navarro, educator and educational psychologist, respectively, systematically analyzed spoken, written, and media narratives encountered by a group of assistant researchers (Danforth & Navarro, 2001). They found that lay people use the concepts and terminology of the DSM ("medical discourse") and that of educators ("school discourse"). From medical discourse, they adopt specific terms, such as "inattention" and "impulsivity," and the tendency to locate pathology in the individual. For example, few speakers identified school as a problem; instead, they endorsed achievement in existing school settings, and attributed difficulties to ADHD-diagnosed individuals. Lay speakers also adopt the clinical focus on negative aspects of individual behavior. For example, of 50 comments concerning individuals taking medication for ADHD, only three framed ADHD-associated behaviors positively. Six media mentions associated ADHD with violence or criminality. In adopting school discourse, people accepted ideals of meritocracy, behavioral conformity, and academic achievement—three areas in which ADHD-diagnosable people often have difficulty. Overall, the authors concluded that lay people's attitudes toward ADHD focused on barriers faced by ADHD-diagnosed people, rather than their strengths.

Danforth and Navarro's data has limitations. It was presumably gathered in the late 1990s, and the assistant researchers collecting commentary were white university students, whose social and media circles were likely limited in some ways. But other, more recent studies also suggest that negative perceptions of ADHD-diagnosed people are prevalent. One research team asked college students to respond to fictional descriptions of people. The students said they would be less likely to want to work with, get to know, or become friends with a person described as having ADHD than they would with a person described as having no disability or minor medical disabilities (Canu, Newman, Morrow, & Pope, 2008). Other researchers surveyed a national sample of youth ages 8 to 18 years. The children and teens responded negatively to vignettes presenting people who had ADHD, speculating that the described person "is more violent" and "gets into trouble more often," although no trouble or violence was included in the vignette (Walker, Coleman, Lee, Squire, & Friesen, 2008). Another study suggests that ADHD-diagnosed children are less well liked than their non-diagnosable peers (Hoza et al., 2005).

How clear is it, though, that the cultural consensus about ADHD shapes these perceptions? Is it more likely that the negative perceptions are based in experience of an intimate's or classmate's intolerable behavior, or of their struggles with work, school, or relationships? Perhaps—but these are not mutually exclusive hypotheses. Both could well be working simultaneously—and they likely are. One way to see this is to consider alternative, less negatively valenced views of ADHD. Psychiatrists Hallowell and Ratey, for example, emphasize positive aspects of ADHD-associated traits and behaviors. In their books intended for nonexpert audiences (for example, Hallowell & Ratey, 2005), they address ADHD-diagnosable individuals with the positive message that having ADHD need not be a burden: "If you don't get help, ADD can curse you and make you wretched. But if you work it right, ADD can enhance your life and make you sparkle" (xxiii).[5] Others suggest that even if people continue to think some ADHD-associated traits and behaviors are undesirable, they could be more tolerant of differences in temperament (McHugh & Kass, 2003; Parens & Johnston, 2009). Similarly, broader definitions of success—or tolerance of failures—are also possible. If these less negative messages prevailed, people's interpretations of many ADHD-associated traits, behavior, and choices could change—and their reactions to ADHD-diagnosed people might as well. The consistently negative portrayals of ADHD instead push the interpretations and reactions toward intolerance.

Byproduct of Practice

Ubiquitous negative portrayals and perceptions of ADHD, like those just discussed, have consistently overwhelmed more positive or tolerant voices. Previous chapters explored the positive feedback loop between science and social needs and interests that reinforces the current, negatively valenced concept of ADHD. Through research and efforts at intervention, ADHD has come to be conceptualized, studied, and managed in particular ways: reinforced intolerance is an unintended byproduct of several patterns in current approaches.

Broadly speaking, familiarity with current ADHD concept in itself contributes to the feedback loop that reinforces ADHD's value valence (see Figure 4.1)—and therefore contributes to the intolerance of ADHD. Familiarity with the associated problems encourages research funding. As data strengthen the correlations of physiological and behavioral differences and associated outcomes with diagnosis, and as research gradually elucidates mechanisms for some features of ADHD, it becomes more natural and accepted to think of people in the value-valenced terms stipulated by the diagnostic criteria. Over time, familiarity helps the category gain power to shape people's views of themselves and of others.

Somewhat more narrowly, scientific concepts and practices contribute (again, inadvertently) to negative perceptions and intolerance. To quickly review, the predominant conception sees ADHD as a biological dysfunction in an individual, dichotomized from "normal" by virtue of focus on differences between "ADHD" and "non-ADHD"; research strategies and priorities reinforce this concept (see Chapter 4). Each of these components (biological, dysfunction, in an individual, dichotomized) contributes to the negative perception of ADHD-diagnosed people, although none is clearly separable from the others nor from elements of cultural context and social and medical practice that also add to the negative perceptions.

Dysfunction

The contribution of conceiving of ADHD as a "dysfunction" does not need more elaboration: Calling something dysfunctional entails perceiving it negatively (*see* Chapters 1 and 4).

Dichotomization

We saw in Chapter 4 that dichotomization establishes a minority group about which people can generalize. Clinically, ADHD is not sharply dichotomized, in that the disorder has fuzzy boundaries (*see* Chapter 1). Yet the dichotomizing tendencies of current science and medicine have for years encouraged perceiving ADHD as importantly different from "normal." For example, when Jensen et al. (2005) write that ADHD-diagnosed people are more likely to experience "...possible justice system contacts and substance abuse troubles, as well as effects on ultimate rates of child abuse, crime, adult mental illness, and accidents with severe injuries" (1628), the words convey significant differences between those who have and do not have ADHD. Because these are not mere differences, but negatively valenced dysfunctions, dichotomization also sharpens the negative portrayal—hence, over time, negative perceptions—of ADHD. Despite the risk of stereotyping, people attribute features of the ADHD category, including the attached values, to individual members of that category. When the category is dichotomized, the negatively valenced attributions have a clearer target.

Biological Views

An often-expressed hope is that biologizing mental illness reduces stigma, by equating mental and physical illness. This argument underlies the American Academy of Child and Adolescent Psychiatry's (AACAP's) ADHD:diabetes analogy. A 2007 press release announced its practice parameter and pocket card on ADHD, stating, "AACAP's Practice Parameter shows that ADHD is a medical illness on par with diabetes or asthma" (Anonymous, 2007). Just as we don't stigmatize those who have diabetes, the argument goes, we should not stigmatize those who have ADHD. But this biologizing strategy is not effective. First, without denying underlying pysiological bases of ADHD, there is an important disanalogy between ADHD and diabetes. Whether a person is sick or healthy, physical attributes are important aspects of a person's self-definition—more so for some than for others. But for many people, what we loosely call "mind" (or "spirit" or "soul," whatever the physical basis of any of these)—along with the decisions, behaviors, conversations, psychological quirks, and other mental phenomena that are subjectively associated with it—hits closer to the "Who is s/he?" question than whether or not their body has a particular physical configuration or disorder. This means that having a dysfunctional mind is not fully analogous to having a dysfunctional pancreas: the former deeply affects *who the person is,* the latter predominantly affects his or her physiology. When it is also understood that the biological dysfunction may be *permanent*—and that it is unlikely to develop in "normals"—this further sharpens the dichotomization, and the normative judgments associated with it.

Medical Care

Ironically, medical care, as practiced today, also contributes to intolerance. One reason for this is that medicine diagnoses and treats individuals, thereby reinforcing the "dysfunction in the individual" view of ADHD. Even when clinicians prefer a contrasting biopsychosocial view, which would place more emphasis on intervening with social context and relations, considerations of cost, time, and sphere of influence usually constrain their practice. Practically speaking, the result is that the primary medical intervention for ADHD is medication.[6]

Medical practice also dichotomizes—of necessity, a patient either gets an ADHD diagnosis or doesn't. This has consequences for clinical care. The dichotomized view of ADHD considers those who are ADHD-diagnosed to be relevantly similar to one another. For example, the clinical practice guidelines in effect through the early 2000s relied on this similarity to make generalized recommendations, downplaying heterogeneity among ADHD-diagnosed individuals (AACAP, 2002; AAP, 2001; Pliszka et al., 2007).[7] For example, the guidelines made few distinctions concerning treatment of the three subtypes of ADHD, or of "pure" ADHD versus ADHD with comorbidity(ies). Guideline authors themselves noted the difficulty: "What is required is information relating specific sociodemographic characteristics (eg, age or sex) or clinical characteristics (eg, subtype of ADHD) to optimal responses to stimulant medication or type of behavior therapy" (American Academy of Pediatrics, 2001, 1041). Good reasons existed—and continue to exist—for this approach: data is limited, the data itself reports generalizations, clinicians need to provide timely assistance, and expert recommendations can facilitate practice. Clinicians are also free to adapt guidelines to individual cases. Still, the similarity of treatment across individuals reinforces dichotomized thinking about the group, among clinicians, patients, and the wider society.

Pharmaceutical treatment, too, has an unintended consequence. Clinicians provide treatment based on medical values such as respect for the blameless status of those suffering from disorders and devotion to treating or curing the sick. Yet the idea that people *can* control certain traits or behaviors with medication, coupled with the negative perceptions of those traits or behaviors, morphs into the idea that people *ought* to do so. The fact that treatment "works" for the most salient manifestations of ADHD strengthens the shift from "can" to "ought." When parents, teachers, and ADHD-diagnosed adults can observe change to behaviors they value, the "ought" of treatment is powerfully reinforced.[8] Providing treatment, and thereby "normalizing" patients' behavior, sends a message that normalization is appropriate—that is, it corroborates intolerance of ADHD.

Power

In U.S. society, science and medicine enjoy high status, ratcheting up the influence of the concepts and practices the fields endorse. Compounding the influence is a power differential between those who are diagnosed—typically, children, adolescents, and adults who are failing to meet social expectations in some way—and the scientists who refine the concept or the clinicians who make the diagnosis. The effect of such influences is only partial—people have many other ways to think about their own or their charges' talents, faults, goals, relationships, and other uniquely combined traits—yet the overall effect reinforces intolerant views of ADHD.

Social Pressures and Practices

Some social pressures are amorphous—critical remarks, annoyed glances, subtle rejections. These, of course, can directly convey intolerant attitudes. Other social pressures contribute to intolerance by institutionalizing narrow definitions of success or normality. Schools and the workplace define success according to "hoops" such as benchmark tests, graduating from successive levels of education, and expectations on annual reviews. Those who struggle with or fail to clear these hurdles, however well or poorly justified the criteria may be, are at a social disadvantage.

The education system and medicine also institutionalize practices intended to help those who need it; concomitantly, they tailor the practices to address social pressures on the institutions of education and medicine. (Such practices are not well established in the workplace.) Schools, committed to each child's success despite large class sizes and limited funding, need quick solutions for children who are struggling or who are difficult to handle in the classroom (see Chapter 3). To provide this, the education system has established practices that tentatively (pending medical diagnosis) identify ADHD-diagnosable children and provide accommodations or support. Medical practice institutionalizes use of generalizations and emphasis on pharmacotherapy (two factors that contribute to intolerance), partly because those practices are cost- and time-minimal, a response to economic pressures on medicine (see Chapter 1). These institutionalized practices dichotomize people into groups that receive and do not receive services, in the process attaching the value valence associated with the two groups. But institutionalization of the practices has the added effect that it makes intolerance of "failure" to achieve benchmarks or exhibition of certain behaviors so matter-of-course that it becomes invisible. Until one questions the definitions of success or criteria for behavior that ground the practices, the intolerance is an accepted routine.

Reification

Many ADHD professionals take the view that "ADHD" is a stand-in for some future, better analysis of human traits, behaviors, or neurophysiology. Even as they use the current concept, they understand it as a heuristic, a social construction, a pragmatic tool, or a hypothesis or model undergoing revision. With these perspectives in view, some experts warn that ADHD should not be reified (Parens & Johnston, 2009)—that is, it should not be prematurely understood as a definitive, clearly identified entity. This is good advice, because avoiding reification has the potential to soften many of the consequences discussed above. For example, it makes less sense to dichotomize "ADHD" and "non-ADHD" if the category is simply a heuristic device; clearly a different heuristic device could create crosscutting categories (see Chapter 6).

Despite the awareness and the warning, however, current language, practice, and portrayal of ADHD all argue that ADHD is typically reified, even by many professionals. For example, when the AACAP states that ADHD is a disease "on a par with diabetes [see above]," they imply that it is a definitive entity, because diabetes is. Teachers and clinicians who recognize, treat, and accommodate ADHD seem to be dealing with an identifiable entity, or their actions make little sense. And, because intolerance depends on having a clearly identified target, it is both a sign and a consequence of ADHD's reification.

In short, these many standard practices take up the negative perceptions of ADHD, institutionalize them, and make them routine. Institutionalized practices, as an accepted norm, have an inertia that makes establishing alternative concepts or practices difficult. The practices thus both naturalize negative perceptions of ADHD and narrow the options for ADHD-diagnosable people.

Effects on Individuals

ADHD-diagnosable people live among the perceptions and practices based on the predominant view of ADHD. The attitudes of others toward their traits and behaviors are part of their everyday experience. The processes of identification, diagnosis, and treatment are directed to them, as are the pressures toward particular forms of behavior control and academic and vocational success. What are the effects? At issue are how individuals perceive the way others think of them, and how their perception of this—along with their own understanding of ADHD—shapes self-image and behavior. The social milieu also powerfully affects the decisions ADHD-diagnosable individuals make for themselves and the choices parents or caregivers make for children.

I do not presume that these effects will be the same for all ADHD-diagnosed or -diagnosable people or for all their caregivers. My portrayal of the effects will ring most true to those who have some doubts about the predominant view of ADHD or about the concepts, perceptions, or practices that affect their own lives or the lives of their families, friends, or acquaintances. Those who endorse society's current norms and expectations—or who at least endorse the necessity of meeting them—and who find treatment acceptable and successful may not agree that they experience intolerance.

Constraints

Institutional structures and policies such as school environments, identification strategies, workplace expectations, health care access, and availability and accessibility of targeted interventions constrain individuals' choices. With the predominant ADHD concept and attendant norms and institutions in place, a parent's decision about how to care for his ADHD-diagnosable child, or an adult's decisions about seeking diagnosis, is very different than it would be in their absence. Established practices are easiest and most available. In contrast, those who question or reject those practices face more difficulty. For example, some parents whose ADHD-diagnosable children do not thrive in current school settings would prefer a change in school environment or expectations to diagnosis and treatment. But alternative schools are not widely available. Similarly, some ADHD-diagnosable adults would prefer different jobs, or different (reasonable) job expectations; again, few options may exist. These constraints, based as they are on particular visions of success, or on particular ways of fitting into the status quo, constitute a key aspect of intolerance; other visions of success or fitting in are less welcome.

The dearth of well-supported treatment options (treatment options that are supported scientifically, clinically, and economically) also constrains choice. Pharmaceutical treatment is the predominant approach in the United States. Between 1991 and 2000, roughly 90% of those receiving an ADHD diagnosis received a prescription for a stimulant (Leslie & Wolraich, 2007; Mayes, Bagwell, & Erkulwater, 2009). More recently, the 2007 AACAP practice parameter (Pliszka et al., 2007) states that for pharmacotherapy without behavior therapy or other intervention (other than psychoeducation) is the first and only treatment necessary for many patients.[9] The parameter also provides much evidence in favor of pharmacotherapy and much against (some favoring) behavior therapy, and it quickly dismisses other proposed forms of treatment or prevention. Very little suggestion of modifying a diagnosed individual's environment is made: One passing reference suggests "additional school resources as appropriate" (902), and the parameter specifies that parents and the ADHD-diagnosed child should receive psychoeducation concerning ADHD (902). This institutionalized focus on drug treatment limits the study and support of behavioral therapy or changes in school or work environments. The resulting lack of options helps explain the sharp increase in the number of stimulant prescriptions for ADHD (*see* Chapter 1).

Social Pressures

ADHD-diagnosed people often feel strong social pressure to succeed relative to the academic, employment, family, or social norms. Failing to live up to these goals or requirements can be painful. Behavioral pediatrician Lawrence Diller says that, in general, ADHD-diagnosed children are happy with their way of being. They may suffer increasingly, though, as they realize that they are not living up to others' expectations (Diller, personal communication, December 17, 2005). Diagnosable adults, too, can feel the pressure. One interpretation calls the uptake of adult ADHD "the medicalization of underachievement" (Conrad & Potter, 2000).

Relatively rigid social, academic, and employment expectations constrain the kind of person it's OK to be. Elliott (2003) points out that even for children, the norms being reinforced are not just standards for childhood and adolescence, such as keeping track of pencils and completing homework and chores. Instead, the worry is also about the child as adult—his or her success in relationships and career. Parents choosing an ADHD diagnosis for their children accept a set of norms for present and future behavior and success that their child struggles with, and with which the parents may or may not wholeheartedly agree. This choice presents difficulties for the child (or for a teen or adult choosing for him- or herself): the chosen standard might either be one they do not endorse, or it might always be out of reach. But the social pressure to achieve the norms can be great, which "...leaves many parents in the unenviable position of either buying into a standard they despise or protesting it through their children" (248).

What standards are inconsistent with those that underlie ADHD diagnosis and treatment? Some alternatives might put less value on standard academic achievement, or give higher status to physical work and play. Another adopts a less mechanistic worldview than the one supporting the predominant concept of ADHD. Mechanistically inclined scientists and clinicians are convinced that much of the distress experienced by ADHD-diagnosable people is (or will be, when the research is further along) traceable to a few specific physiological dysfunction(s). But this conception is shared only in part with other communities. Members of some scientific and clinical communities doubt that mechanistic explanations and interventions can substitute for higher-level approaches to helping people cope with social or emotional struggles. In these alternative views, biopsychosocial, psychoanalytic, cognitive, behavioral, or other models of mental disorder should ground clinical practice. Others—often, but not exclusively, "lay" people or members of religious communities—reject mechanistic thinking on the grounds that it dissolves meaning, and the intangible properties and significance people assign to meaning. In particular, those who do not adopt a mechanistic worldview are concerned that it privileges the measurable, while trivializing immeasurables such as self-concept or relationships.

For example, some religious communities consider the intangibles of faith, mystery, and morality at least as valuable as the conclusions of mechanistic science or its clinical partners. Psychiatrist Paul McHugh, speaking of the medicalization of human behavior, describes one of the fundamental conflicts between a mechanistic and a Christian perspective:

> You define "medicalization" as that view reducing all forms of human distress and disorder to aspects of "sickness", expressions of "patient-hood" and thus expressly open to technical, mostly bio-medical, correction at the hands of experts for whom ideas of good and evil, freedom and responsibility, sanctity and sin, approval and reprobation are meaningless. Medicalization is a materialist ethos with roots in both biological sciences and contemporary medicine (McHugh & Kass, 2003, unpaginated).

McHugh does not deny the benefits of science in general or neuroscience in particular. For example, he specifies that he uses psychopharmaceuticals judiciously in his practice. But he does portray the "materialist ethos" as preference for mechanism over meaning, and as perpetuating a fundamentally flawed view of humans and human distress. ADHD-diagnosable people who hold this standard—or one of many other alternatives—may find it difficult to accept mainstream recommendations.

Relief, Ambivalence, Acceptance

But for those who agree with the norms embedded in ADHD concepts and practice, diagnosis and treatment can come as a welcome relief. Adults dismayed with broken relationships, lack of success at work, or past or present academic failures often embrace the biomedical interpretation of their life story. Media portrayals, at least in the 1990s, tended to present diagnosis in this light (Schmitz, Filippone, & Edelman, 2003). Even in the case of agreement, though, relief may only be one aspect of an individual's reaction. A small (eight participants) qualitative study of adults found that relief was the first of six stages of adaptation to diagnosis and treatment (Young, Bramham, Gray, & Rose, 2008). Next, the participants experienced confusion, anger, grief, and anxiety as they worked through what they perceived as lost opportunities and misunderstandings prior to their diagnosis. Finally, seven of the eight accommodated and accepted the diagnosis; the eighth stopped taking medication. Although coming to terms with diagnosis and treatment was not easy, in the end this group considered it a net benefit. Notably, however, even after acceptance, the participants remained anxious about the stigma associated with diagnosis.

Agreeing with the norms may also be a matter of degree, ambivalence, or pragmatism. According to Ilina Singh, many parents making medication decisions for their children waffle uneasily between perspectives, at times justifying drug use, at other times justifying withholding a dose (Singh, 2005). These parents may be weighing competing goals for their children's behavior—for example, compliance versus spontaneity—finding one more valuable in one situation, one in another (Litton, 2005). Parents, and ADHD-diagnosed adults, may also prioritize pragmatism: They may simply want to make their children's lives, or their own, easier or more explicable in the most straightforward way available. The choices, though, cannot be abstracted from the social norms and institutional constraints that structure them. Via the norms and constraints, intolerance affects even those with positive views of social institutions, diagnosis, or treatment.

Internalizing

An important effect of diagnosis and treatment is that people may come to view themselves as exemplifying their diagnostic category. Philosopher Ian Hacking has described this as part of a looping effect (Hacking, 1995); some sociologists and psychologists study a similar phenomenon under the general concept of "labeling theory" or "social representations theory." According to Hacking's analysis, scientists (and others) identify certain "kinds" of people, singling out single out certain traits, propensities, or life stories as marking significant categories. Two of his examples are "child abuse" and "teen-age pregnancy." Each category provides the opportunity for "kinds" that did not exist earlier in history—people in earlier generations hit children, but they were not thought of, nor did they consider themselves, child abusers; adolescents became pregnant, but the requisite norms of marriage and delayed maternity that raise concern about young mothers did not, until recently, elicit the description "teen-age pregnancy." In Hacking's view, people identify the kinds for the purpose of intervention. Labeling an individual as a certain kind also confers a moral status: it may be criminalized, as in the case of the child abuser, or may be medicalized, as for the pregnant teenager. The "looping effect" occurs when individuals categorize themselves according to the labels and begin to act in accordance with the labels. Others also reconstitute their image of those individuals, altering their behavior toward those categorized. Going beyond labeling theory, however, Hacking says that this step makes possible new scientific knowledge of the kind. The knowledge changes the kind, further altering self-perceptions and views of others toward those affected.

That the kinds are biologized, Hacking has noted, does not vitiate the looping effects. Someone who believes him- or herself to have a biological dysfunction will behave differently than one who believes him- or herself to have (for example) a moral failing.

In the case of ADHD, internalizing the predominant view entails accepting the core features of that category: one's biology is dysfunctional, and it is unlike that of the majority; one's social, academic, or employment difficulties result at least in part from this difference, and to that extent *not* from others in relationship or from school or work circumstances. In these and other ways, internalizing involves understanding oneself in relation to the criteria and values embedded in the category.

Singh concluded from a qualitative study that 8- to 12-year-old ADHD-diagnosed children had an emerging sense of self that was in part structured according to their ADHD diagnosis (Singh, 2007). As the author cautions, it is important not to overgeneralize these results, as this was a pilot study involving only 20 boys and 3 girls, with the sample importantly limited to white children in the United Kingdom. Yet the interviews were suggestive: For example, the children thought of themselves as "good" and more "normal" when taking Ritalin and "bad" when not. They did not think that Ritalin use transformed their "badness," however; they felt that "badness" persisted as a core dimension of their character. They said they were sad about their inability to control themselves at times and expressed worry at what others thought of them.

Singh observes that the children described their experience in binaries—good/bad, normal/abnormal, happy/sad. She suggests that the binaries may represent either cognitive immaturity or, more likely, an artifact of the way the questions were presented. She observes as well that the children might have gleaned their moral view of their own character from interactions with their caregivers. An alternative interpretation is that the children have, with fair accuracy, internalized (a term I equate here with Singh's structuring of the emerging sense of self) the predominant biomedical view of their own condition. The binary conception corresponds to its dichotomized view; the bad/abnormal/sad an internalization of the embedded values. It also seems the internalizing may be reluctant; although the children reported satisfaction with being more "normal" when taking Ritalin, they also said that they were happier when off medication, and sad when taking it.

Again, it is important not to overplay this single study. Not only is there a limited and nondiverse sample, but it is also important to know how non-diagnosed but diagnosable children view themselves. This information would help decide between two hypotheses: On the one hand, internalizing the diagnosis might lead to the children's binaries and the moral expressions; on the other, internalizing more general features of the social environment—such as its use of binaries and moral expressions—might engender the children's way of thinking.[10]

It is at least unambiguous that the symptoms associated with ADHD are disvalued and that the ADHD category is a powerful one—salient, clear, much-discussed, overt, and persistent. And of course, the very point of diagnosis and treatment is to tamp down the symptoms—to change the way a person thinks and behaves. It is hard to imagine, given this, that diagnosis would leave self-image unaffected.

Why Uptake, Then?

If accepting the diagnosis really means bowing to social pressures and constraints, and internalizing negative self-perceptions, the widespread uptake of ADHD seems paradoxical. Why would such large numbers actively seek diagnosis and treatment for themselves or their children (Sax & Kautz, 2003)? The social pressures, practices, and institutions already discussed go a long way toward answering this question; given these, diagnosis and treatment are often the best option available. Speaking theoretically, it seems that people must weigh a trade-off. They, or their children, face intolerance of their ADHD-type traits and behaviors *with or without* a diagnosis. Without a diagnosis, they can avoid the permanence, biologizing, and stereotyping that come with the label—but they get no assistance. With a diagnosis, they get the opposite. This means that the perceived value of assistance is likely to play a major role in the decision. If one endorses (or acquiesces to) valuing the forms of control, focused attention, and detail orientation facilitated by treatment, then treatment may make a positive difference. Associated as these forms of control are with long-term goals of academic, occupational, and social achievement, the expected tangible rewards are often great enough to outweigh worries about the choice.[11]

Nevertheless, in the case of children, who typically do not request diagnosis and treatment for themselves, the decision of others to make the request involves intolerance of a child's behavior—even if the decision is made because the parents, teachers, physicians, and others involved sincerely believe that the change is for the best in the long run...and even if they are right, according to their chosen criteria. This is because the social system in which the choice is "right" is one that in principle could be changed, allowing a different response to the child's behavior, or a different set of criteria to assess it. For adults, who do typically request diagnosis and treatment, the intolerance issue is murkier. But many of the adults who choose diagnosis and treatment are constrained in their choice, given their relative powerlessness or vulnerability and the intolerance of their traits in relationships and in the workplace. For them, as for parents making treatment decisions for their children, their hand may well be forced.

The Drug Wars and Skeptics' Intolerance

The long-lasting backlash to the predominant view of ADHD provides alternative concepts and management options.[12] The wide range of counterviews draws on multiple values, especially different perspectives on the appropriate definitions and relative importance of liberty, responsibility, and individualism. But the backlash can also pressure ADHD-diagnosable people. The pressure often comes in the form of a contradicting "ought"—rather than seeking diagnosis and treatment, a diagnosable person (or parent of a diagnosable child) ought to reject it. Like the predominant view, the alternatives are typically based on concern for diagnosable people.[13] Yet some of the positions present intransigence about choice that—given the limited options available—can rise to a level of intolerance.

Some opponents' claims are extreme.[14] For example, the deeply skeptical psychiatrist Thomas Szasz writes, "The history of psychiatry is the history of 'ethical psychiatric services,' as psychiatrists and the society in which they have lived defined what was ethical. Euthanasia of crippled children and mental patients was an ethical psychiatric service in Nazi Germany...and so is giving Ritalin to five million children" (Schaler, 2004, 325). Elsewhere, Szasz explains his view of the link: The medical field is a coercive, paternalistic instrument of state control. "The engine that drives the psychiatrist's proclivity for coercive paternalism and aversion to liberty and responsibility is his deep-seated love of 'liberalism,' that is, his bias for statism of the leftist totalitarian type" (Schaler, 2004, 108). Psychiatrist Peter Breggin, in his book *Talking Back to Ritalin,* avers, "We are raising a generation of children, many of whom are being told they have something wrong in their brains that won't ever go away...Many of them understand that they have been given pills instead of love, understanding, or attention" (Breggin, 1998). Such views have enough influence that they have not disappeared, despite the continued increase in rates of diagnosis and treatment. If family or friends of an ADHD-diagnosable person adopt one of these stances, they may complicate an already difficult decision about diagnosis or treatment.

Less hyperbolic concerns about overdiagnosis or overmedication draw on some of the same themes. A more moderate version of Szaszian themes is to think that the predominant view limits liberty (is coercive) when it holds too strict a view of normality—in a toned-down view, medical practice *may* do this, but it is a matter of degree. McHugh, for example, values individual variation, objecting to a goal of "normalization" through pharmacotherapy that unnecessarily obscures or undermines features of individuals.[15] When medical practice describes difference as disorder, and assumes that a "twisted neuron" (neurological dysfunction) is the cause, what gets left out are elements of an individual's "unique and special form of life" (McHugh & Kass, 2003, unpaginated). McHugh argues that medication is sometimes valuable but that decreasing differences may overstep important bounds.

Others think that the key problem is overemphasis on the individual at the expense of recognizing the role of environment on shaping and intervening in ADHD symptoms. Such "environmentalists" reason that the focus on drug treatment is misdirected, in that it tends to downplay possibilities such as altering the school, occupational, or other environments in which the individual works or plays. British child and adolescent psychiatrist Sami Timimi is a thoroughgoing environmentalist concerning ADHD. In his view, "...the origins of the current epidemic of ADHD lies deep in cultural machinery of Western society" (Timimi, 2005, 146), rather than within the individual. He opts to work with families to look for a "holistic, integrated, multi-perspective model" (147) that emphasizes environment, family, and common-sense solutions to behavioral problems.

Proponents of medication use sometimes suggest that medication allows people to take responsibility for work, school, and personal affairs by making it easier for them to do so. Timimi and McHugh, in contrast, both worry about medication undermining a sense of responsibility. Part of Timimi's concern about ADHD medication is that, "...in the long term you create a group of children who are dependent (on the drugs and on the doctors who prescribe them)..." (147). The children do not learn to manage their own behavior, instead relying on medication. McHugh agrees that some diagnoses, including adult ADD (*see* endnote 5), help people shelter themselves from responsibilities by providing an excuse for failures to meet them.

Similar motivations stimulate concern about overdiagnosis. Professionals who place a higher value on liberty, responsibility, or individual variation than on assistance would tend to judge fewer people to "have ADHD" than those who reverse the relative ranking. A higher tolerance for individual variation might mean, for example, that a rater would be less likely to say a child met diagnostic criteria, such as being "often" distracted by "extraneous" stimuli, or "often" talking "excessively" (American Psychiatric Association, 2000, 92–93). A diagnostician placing a higher premium on assuming drug- and diagnosis-free responsibility for one's actions would require more disability before allowing an affected individual the "excuse" of a diagnosis. One who placed a high value on liberty would raise the bar for interference by a third party. Overdiagnosis, in these views, means that the bar for diagnosis is set too low, based on these criteria.

Depending on how such concerns are taken up and communicated among family, friends, and the wider society, they may open options for ADHD-diagnosable people, or they may add layers of guilt or worry. It is one thing to say, "ADHD is just an excuse," and quite another to teach and encourage responsible behavior. It is one thing to suggest alternatives when a family is in a position to provide them, and quite another when they are not. When doubts about drug use or overdiagnosis wax dogmatic, versions of intolerance result. The range of non-mainstream values and expectations that drive these versions push diagnosable people (or diagnosable children's parents) in various directions, but generally away from diagnosis and pharmacotherapy. Although these views are not dominant at present, they are a part of the social milieu that many have to negotiate.

Conclusion

At present, the predominant view of ADHD, and the accidental intolerance associated with it, has the upper hand. The complex mix of the needs and interests of science, medicine, education, employers, government, the pharmaceutical industry, families, and individuals has reached a consensus that teaches us to perceive and react to ADHD according to that predominant view. Unfortunately, because of the much-reinforced negative valence of the ADHD category, our perceptions and reactions are clouded by intolerance.

Admittedly, the term "intolerance" is loaded. Certainly, it is not the *intention* of the vast majority of professionals, parents, or others involved with ADHD to promote or accept intolerance. Quite the contrary—many experts in the field lobby against stigmatization of ADHD, and at least some of the concepts and practices surrounding ADHD also embed compassion for ADHD-diagnosable individuals. Still, negative perceptions and the dearth of options are a fact of life for diagnosable people. Until the perceptions can be effectively dispersed, and options opened, "intolerance" is an apt term. The question then becomes, what do we do about it? That is the subject of the concluding chapter.

REFERENCES

Abikoff, H. B., Hechtman, L., Klein, R. G., Gallagher, R., Fleiss, K., Etcovitch, J., et al. (2004). Social functioning in children with ADHD treated with long-term methylphenidate and multimodal psychosocial treatment. *Journal of the American Academy of Child and Adolescent Psychiatry, 43*(7), 820–829.

Alban-Metcalfe, J., Cheng-Lai, A., & Ma, T. (2002). Teacher and student teacher ratings of attention-deficit/hyperactivity disorder in three cultural settings. *International Journal of Disability, Development and Education, 49*(3), 281–299.

American Academy of Child and Adolescent Psychiatry (2002). AACAP Official Action: Practice parameter for the use of stimulant medications in the treatment of children, adolescents, and adults. *Journal of the American Academy of Child and Adolescent Psychiatry, 41*(Suppl 2), 26S–49S.

American Academy of Pediatrics, Committee on Quality Improvement, Subcommittee on Attention-Deficit/Hyperactivity Disorder (2001). Clinical practice guideline: treatment of the school-aged child with attention-deficit/hyperactivity disorder. *Pediatrics, 108*(4), 1033–1044.

American Psychiatric Association (2000). *Diagnostic and Statistical Manual of Mental Disorders* (4, Text Revision ed.). Arlington, VA: American Psychiatric Association.

Angell, M. (2004). *The Truth About the Drug Companies: How They Deceive Us and What to Do About It*. New York: Random House.

Anonymous (2004). Economic impact of ADHD. Retrieved June 17, 2005, from http://www.medicalnewstoday.com/medicalnews.php?newsid=13210

Anonymous (2005a). *Medical Crossfire: Special Edition: Assessing the Safety of ADHD Medications: An Expert Panel Considers the Clinical Significance of Potential Adverse Effects*. (Vol. 6, pp. 1–21). New Brunswick, NJ: University of Medicine and Dentistry of New Jersey and Liberty Communications Network.

Anonymous (2005b). $77 billion in lost income is attributed to ADHD annually in the United States (May 23, 2005). Retrieved June 17, 2005, from http://www.eurekalert.org/pub_releases/2005-05/pn-bi051905.php.

Anonymous (2007). AACAP introduces new ADHD practice parameter and pocketcard Retrieved April 29, 2008, from http://www.aacap.org/cs/2007_press_releases/aacap_introduces_new_adhd_practice_parameter_and_pocketcard

Arnold, L. E. (1996). Sex differences in ADHD: Conference summary. *Journal of Abnormal Child Psychology, 24*(5), 555–569.

Aronson, L. J. (1971). The psychologist and minimal brain dysfunction: ten steps to maximum incompetence. *Mental Hygiene, 55*(4), 523–525.

Baird, J., Stevenson, J. C., & Williams, D. C. (2000). The evolution of ADHD: a disorder of communication? *The Quarterly Review of Biology, 75*(1), 17–35.

Barkley, R. A. (1997). *ADHD and the Nature of Self-Control*. New York: The Guilford Press.

Barkley, R. A., Murphy, K. R., & Kwasnik, D. (1996). Motor vehicle driving competencies and risks in teens and young adults with attention deficit hyperactivity disorder. *Pediatrics, 98*(6), 1089–1095.

Barry, T. D., Lyman, R. D., & Klinger, L. G. (2002). Academic underachievement and attention-deficit/hyperactivity disorder: the negative impact of symptom severity on school performance. *Journal of School Psychology, 40*(3), 259–283.

Bastiaansen, D., Koot, H. M., Ferdinand, R. F., & Verhulst, F. C. (2004). Quality of life in children with psychiatric disorders: Self-, parent, and clinician report. *Journal of the American Academy of Child and Adolescent Psychiatry, 43*(2), 221–230.

Biederman, J., & Faraone, S. V. (2006). The Effects of Attention-Deficit/Hyperactivity Disorder on Employment and Household Income. *Medscape General Medicine, 8*(3), 12. Retrieved September 7, 2007, from http://www.medscape.com/viewarticle/536264

Birnbaum, H. G., Kessler, R. C., Lowe, S. W., Secnik, K., Greenberg, P. E., Leong, S. A., et al. (2005). Costs of attention-deficit hyperactivity disorder (ADHD) in the US: Excess costs of persons with ADHD and their family members in 2000. *Current Medical Research and Opinion, 21*(2), 195–206.

Brand, S., Dunn, R., & Greb, F. (2002). Learning styles of students with attention deficit hyperactivity disorder: who are they and how can we teach them? *The Clearing House, 75*(5), 268–273.

Breggin, P. R. (1998). *Talking Back to Ritalin: What Doctors Aren't Telling You About Stimulants for Children*. Monroe, ME: Common Courage Press.

Brewis, A. (2002). Social and biological measures of hyperactivity and inattention: are they describing similar underlying constructs of child behavior? *Social Biology, 49*(1–2), 99–115.

Broudy, H. S. (1976). Ideological, political, and moral considerations in the use of drugs in hyperkinetic therapy. *School Review, 85*(1), 43–60.

Bussing, R., Gary, F. A., Mills, T. L., & Garvan, C. W. (2003). Parental explanatory models of ADHD: Gender and cultural variations. *Social Psychiatry and Psychiatric Epidemiology, 38*, 563–575.

Bussing, R., Gary, F. A., Mills, T. L., & Garvan, C. W. (2003). Parental explanatory models of ADHD: gender and cultural variations. *Social Psychiatry & Psychiatric Epidemiology, 38*(10), 563–575.

Canu, W. H., Newman, M. L., Morrow, T. L., & Pope, D. L. W. (2008). Social appraisal of adult ADHD: Stigma and influences of the beholder's Big Five personality traits. *Journal of Attention Disorders, 11*, 700–710.

Castellanos, F. X., Lee, P. P., Sharp, W., Jeffries, N. O., Greenstein, D. K., Clasen, L. S., et al. (2002). Developmental trajectories of brain volume abnormalities in children and adolescents with attention-deficit/hyperactivity disorder. *JAMA, 288*(14), 1740–1748.

Chen, M., Seipp, C. M., & Johnston, C. (2008). Mothers' and fathers' attributions and beliefs in families of girls and boys with attention-deficit/hyperactivity disorder. [References]. *Child Psychiatry & Human Development, 39*(1), 85–99.

Christakis, D. A., Zimmerman, F. J., DiGiuseppe, D. L., & McCarty, C. A. (2004). Early television exposure and subsequent attentional problems in children. *Pediatrics, 113*(4), 708–713.

Clarke, A. R., Barry, R. J., McCarthy, R., Selikowitz, M., & Johnstone, S. J. (2007). Effects of stimulant medications on the EEG of girls with attention-deficit/hyperactivity disorder. *Clinical Neurophysiology, 118,* 2700–2708.

Cohn, H. D. (1971). Methylphenidate and minimal brain dysfunction (letter). *The New England Journal of Medicine, 285*(20), 1150.

Conrad, P., & Potter, D. (2000). From hyperactive child to ADHD adults: observations on the expansion of medical categories. *Social Problems, 47*(4), 559–582.

Danforth, S., & Navarro, V. (2001). Hyper talk: sampling the social construction of ADHD in everyday language. *Anthropology and Education Quarterly, 32*(2), 167–190.

Davison, J. C. (2001). Attention deficit/hyperactivity disorder: perspectives of participants in the identification and treatment process. *Journal of Educational Thought, 35*(3), 227–247.

Derks, E. M., Hudziak, J. J., & Boomsma, D. I. (2007). Why more boys than girls with ADHD receive treatment: a study of Dutch twins. *Twin Res Hum Genet, 10*(5), 765–770.

Diller, L. (2005). Bitter Pill: Ritalin and the growing influence of big pharma. *Psychotherapy Networker, 29*(1), unpaginated.

Dimoska, A., Johnstone, S. J., Barry, R. J., & Clarke, A. R. (2003). Inhibitory motor control in children with attention-deficit/hyperactivity disorder: event-related potentials in the stop-signal paradigm. *Biological Psychiatry, 54,* 1345–1354.

Ding, Y.-C., Chi, H.-C., Grady, D. L., Morishima, A., Kidd, J. R., Kidd, K. K., et al. (2002). Evidence of positive selection acting at the human dopamine receptor D4 gene locus. *PNAS, 99*(1), 309–314.

DiScala, C., Lescohier, I., Barthel, M., & Li, G. (1998). Injuries to children with attention deficit hyperactivity disorder. *Pediatrics, 102*(6), 1415–1421.

Durston, S., Pol, H. E. H., Schnack, H. G., Buitelaar, J. K., Steenhuis, M. P., Minderaa, R. B., et al. (2004). Magnetic resonance imaging of boys with attention-deficit/hyperactivity disorder and their unaffected siblings. *Journal of the American Academy of Child and Adolescent Psychiatry, 43*(3), 332–340.

Eisenberg, L. (1972). Symposium: behavior modification by drugs. III. The clinical use of stimulant drugs in children. *Pediatrics, 49*(5), 709–715.

Elliott, C. (2000). Pursued by Happiness and Beaten Senseless: Prozac and the American Dream. *Hastings Center Report, 30*(2), 7–12.

Elliott, C. (2003). *Better Than Well: American Medicine Meets the American Dream.* New York: W. W. Norton & Company.

Flood, W. A., & Wilder, D. A. (2002). Antecedent assessment and assessment-based treatment of off-task behavior in a child diagnosed with attention deficit-hyperactivity disorder (ADHD). *Education and Treatment of Children, 25*(3), 331–338.

Freeman, R. D. (1976). Minimal brain dysfunction, hyperactivity, and learning disorders: epidemic or episode? *School Review, 85*(1), 5–29.

Gaub, M., & Carlson, C. L. (1997). Gender differences in ADHD: A meta-analysis and critical review. *Journal of the American Academy of Child & Adolescent Psychiatry, 36*(8), 1036–1045.

Graetz, B. W., Sawyer, M. G., & Baghurst, P. (2005). Gender differences among children with DSM-IV ADHD in Australia. *Journal of the American Academy of Child & Adolescent Psychiatry, 44*(2), 159–168.

Greene, R. W., Biederman, J., Faraone, S. V., Monuteaux, M. C., Mick, E., DuPre, E. P., et al. (2001). Social impairment in girls with ADHD: patterns, gender comparisons, and correlates. *Journal of the American Academy of Child & Adolescent Psychiatry, 40*(6), 704–710.

Gresham, F. M., Lane, K. L., & Lambros, K. M. (2000). Comorbidity of conduct problems and ADHD: identification of "fledgling psychopaths." *Journal of Emotional and Behavioral Disorders, 8*(2), 83–93.

Grinspoon, L., & Singer, S. B. (1973). Amphetamines in the treatment of hyperkinetic children. *Harvard Educational Review, 43*(4), 515–555.

Hackett, R. (1975). In praise of praise. *American Education, 11*, 11–15.

Hacking, I. (1995). The looping effects of human kinds. In D. P. Sperber, D; Premack, AJ (Ed.), *Causal Cognition: A Multidisciplinary Debate* (pp. 351–383). Oxford, England: Clarendon Press.

Hallowell, E. M., & Ratey, J. J. (2005). *Delivered From Distraction: Getting the Most out of Life with Attention Deficit Disorder*. New York: Ballantine Books.

Hechtman, L., Abikoff, H. B., Klein, R. G., Weiss, G., Respitz, C., Kouri, J., et al. (2004). Academic achievement and emotional status of children with ADHD treated with long-term methylphenidate and multimodal psychosocial treatment. *Journal of the American Academy of Child and Adolescent Psychiatry, 43*(7), 812–819.

Hinshaw, S. P., Carte, E. T., Fan, C., Jassy, J. S., & Owens, E. B. (2007). Neuropsychological functioning of girls with attention-deficit/hyperactivity disorder followed prospectively into adolescence: evidence for continuing deficits? *Neuropsychology, 21*(2), 263–273.

Hoza, B., Mrug, S., Gerdes, A. C., Bukowski, W. M., Kraemer, H. C., Wigal, T., et al. (2005). What aspects of peer relationships are impaired in children with attention-deficit/hyperactivity disorder? *Journal of Consulting and Clinical Psychology, 73*(3), 411–423.

Jensen, P. S., Garcia, J. A., Glied, S., Crowe, M., Foster, M., Schlander, M., et al. (2005). Cost-effectiveness of ADHD treatments: Findings from the Multimodal

Treatment Study of Children with ADHD. *American Journal of Psychiatry, 162*(9), 1628–1636.

Kenny, T. J., Clemmens, R. L., Hudson, B. W., Lentz, G., A., Jr., Cicci, R., Nair, P. (1971). Characteristics of children referred because of hyperactivity. *The Journal of Pediatrics, 79*(4), 618–622.

Krauch, V. (1971). Hyperactive engineering. *American Education, 7*, 12–16.

Leibson, C. L., Katusic, S. K., Barbaresi, W. J., Ransom, J., & O'Brien, P. C. (2001). Use and costs of medical care for children and adolescents with and without attention-deficit/hyperactivity disorder. *JAMA, 285*(1), 60–66.

Leslie, L. K., & Wolraich, M. L. (2007). ADHD service use patterns in youth. *Ambul Pediatr, 7*(1 Suppl), 107–120.

Levy, F., Hay, D. A., Bennett, K. S., & McStephen, M. (2005). Gender Differences in ADHD Subtype Comorbidity. [References]. *Journal of the American Academy of Child & Adolescent Psychiatry, 44*(4), 368–376.

Litton, P. (2005). ADHD, values, and the self. *American Journal of Bioethics, 5*(3), 65–67.

Madras, B. K., Miller, G. M., & Fischman, A. J. (2002). The dopamine transporter: relevance to attention deficit hyperactivity disorder (ADHD). *Behavioural Brain Research, 130*, 57–63.

Mayes, R., Bagwell, C., & Erkulwater, J. (2009). *Medicating Children: ADHD and Pediatric Mental Health*. Cambridge, MA: Harvard University Press.

McHugh, P. (1999). How Psychiatry Lost Its Way. *Commentary, 108*(5), 32–38.

McHugh, P., & Kass, L. R. (2003). Exchange of Letters on Medicalization Between Leon R. Kass, M.D. and Paul McHugh, M.D. Retrieved January 2, 2006, from http://www.bioethics.gov/background/kass_mchugh.html

McNeil Consumer & Specialty Pharmaceuticals: ADHD Success Stories on DVD: Once-Daily Concerta (methylphenidate HCl) (2003). [DVD]. Fort Washington, PA: McNeil-PPC, Inc.

Miller, F. (1973). Getting Billy into the game. *American Education, 9*, 22–27.

Molina, B. S. G., Flory, K., Hinshaw, S. P., Greiner, A. R., Arnold, L. E., Swanson, J. M., et al. (2007). Delinquent behavior and emerging substance use in the MTA at 36 months: prevalence, course, and treatment effects. *Journal of the American Academy of Child and Adolescent Psychiatry, 46*(8), 1028–1040.

MTA Cooperative Group (2004a). National Institute of Mental Health multimodal treatment study of ADHD follow-up: 24-month outcomes of treatment strategies for attention-deficit/hyperactivity disorder. *Pediatrics, 113*(4), 754–761.

MTA Cooperative Group (2004b): National Institute of Mental Health multimodal treatment study of ADHD follow-up: changes in effectiveness and growth after the end of treatment. *Pediatrics, 113*(4), 762–769.

Newcorn, J. H., Halperin, J. M., Jensen, P. S., Abikoff, H. B., Arnold, L. E., Cantwell, D. P., et al. (2001). Symptom profiles in children with ADHD: effects of comorbidity and gender. *Journal of the American Academy of Child and Adolescent Psychiatry, 40*(2), 137–146.

Novik, T. S., Hervas, A., Ralston, S. J., Dalsgaard, S., Rodrigues Pereira, R., & Lorenzo, M. J. (2006). Influence of gender on attention-deficit/hyperactivity disorder in Europe—ADORE. *Eur Child Adolesc Psychiatry, 15 Suppl 1*, 115–124.

Ohan, J. L., & Johnston, C. (2005). Gender Appropriateness of Symptom Criteria for Attention-Deficit/Hyperactivity Disorder, Oppositional-Defiant Disorder, and Conduct Disorder. [References]. *Child Psychiatry & Human Development, 35*(4), 359–381.

Ohan, J. L., & Johnston, C. (2007). What is the social impact of ADHD in girls? A multi-method assessment. *J Abnorm Child Psychol, 35*(2), 239–250.

Parens, E., & Johnston, J. (2009). Facts, values, and Attention-Deficit Hyperactivity Disorder (ADHD): an update on the controversies. *Child Adolesc Psychiatry Ment Health, 3*(1), 1.

Pliszka, S., Bernet, W., Bukstein, O., Walter, H. J., Arnold, V., Beitchman, J., et al. (2007). Practice parameter for the assessment and treatment of children and adolescents with attention-deficit/hyperactivity disorder *Journal of the American Academy of Child and Adolescent Psychiatry, 46*(7), 894–921.

Purdie, N., Hattie, J., & Carroll, A. (2002). A review of the research on interventions for attention deficit hyperactivity disorder: what works best? *Review of Educational Research, 72*(1), 61–99.

Quinn, P., & Wigal, S. (2004). Perceptions of girls and ADHD: results from a national survey. *Medgenmed [Computer File]: Medscape General Medicine, 6*(2):2, unpaginated.

Quinn, P. O. (2005). Treating Adolescent Girls and Women With ADHD: Gender-Specific Issues. [References]. *Journal of Clinical Psychology, 61*(5), 579–587.

Renstrom, R. (1976). The teacher and the social worker in stimulant drug treatment of hyperactive children. *School Review, 85*(1), 97–108.

Robin, S. S., & Bosco, J. J. (1976). The social context of stimulant drug treatment for hyperkinetic children. *School Review, 85*(1), 141–154.

Sax, L., & Kautz, K. J. (2003). Who first suggests the diagnosis of attention-deficit/hyperactivity disorder? *Annals of Family Medicine, 1*(3), 171–174.

Schaler, J. A. (Ed.). (2004). *Szasz Under Fire: The Psychiatric Abolitionist Faces His Critics* (Vol. 1). Chicago: Open Court.

Schirduan, V., Case, K., & Faryniarz, J. (2002). How ADHD students are smart. *The Educational Forum, 66*(4), 324–328.

Schmitz, M. F., Filippone, P., & Edelman, E. M. (2003). Social representations of attention deficit/hyperactivity disorder, 1988–1997. *Culture $ Psychology, 9*(4), 383–406.

Schulte, F. J. (1971). Current concepts in minimal brain dysfunction (editorial). *JAMA, 217*(9), 1237–1238.

Singh, I. (2003). Boys will be boys: Fathers' perspectives on ADHD symptoms, diagnosis, and drug treatment. *Harvard Review of Psychiatry, 11*(6), 308–316.

Singh, I. (2005). Will the "real boy" please behave: Dosing dilemmas for parents of boys with ADHD. *The American Journal of Bioethics, 5*(3), 34–47.

Singh, I. (2007). Clinical implications of ethical concepts: moral self-understandings in children taking methylphenidate for ADHD. *Clin Child Psychol Psychiatry, 12*(2), 167–182.

Solanto, M. V., Arnsten, A. F. T., & Castellanos, F. X. (2001). *Stimulant Drugs and ADHD: Basic and Clinical Neuroscience.* Oxford: Oxford University Press.

Sourander, A., Elonheimo, H., Niemela, S., Nuutila, A. M., Helenius, H., Sillanmaki, L., et al. (2006). Childhood predictors of male criminality: a prospective population-based follow-up study from age 8 to late adolescence. *J Am Acad Child Adolesc Psychiatry, 45*(5), 578–586.

Steger, J., Imhof, K., Steinhausen, H.-C., & al, e. (2000). Brain mapping of bilateral interactions in attention deficit hyperactivity disorder and control boys. *Clinical Neurophysiology, 111,* 1141–1156.

Stewart, M. A. (1976). Is hyperactivity abnormal? and other unanswered questions. *School Review, 85*(1), 31–42.

Stinnett, T. A., Crawford, S. A., Gillespie, M. D., Cruce, M. K., & Langford, C. A. (2001). Factors affecting treatment acceptability for psychostimulant medication versus psychoeducational intervention. *Psychology in the Schools, 38*(6), 585–591.

Swanson, J., Oosterlaan, J., Murias, M., Schuck, S., Flodman, P., Spence, M. A., et al. (2000). Attention deficit/hyperactivity disorder children with a 7-repeat allele of the dopamine receptor D4 gene have extreme behavior but normal performance on critical neuropsychological tests of attention. *PNAS, 97*(9), 4754–4759.

Teicher, M. H., Anderson, C. M., Polcari, A., Glod, C. A., Maas, L. C., Renshaw, P. F. (2000). Functional deficits in basal ganglia of children with attention-deficit/hyperactivity disorder shown with functional magnetic resonance imaging relaxometry. *Nature Medicine, 6*(4), 470–473.

Thurber, J. R., Heller, T. L., & Hinshaw, S. P. (2002). The social behaviors and peer expectation of girls with attention deficit hyperactivity disorder and comparison girls. [References]. *Journal of Clinical Child and Adolescent Psychology, 31*(4), 443–452.

Timimi, S. (2005). *Naughty Boys: Anti-Social Behaviour, ADHD and the Role of Culture.* Houndmills, UK: Palmgrave Macmillan.

Towbin, A. (1971). Organic causes of minimal brain dysfunction: perinatal origin of minimal cerebral lesions. *JAMA, 217*(9), 1207–1214.

Walker, J. S., Coleman, D., Lee, J., Squire, P. N., & Friesen, B. J. (2008). Children's stigmatization of childhood depression and ADHD: magnitude and demographic variation in a national sample. *Journal of the American Academy of Child and Adolescent Psychiatry, 47*(8), 912–920.

Wikler, A., Dixon, J. F., & Parker, J. B. (1970). Brain function in problem children and controls: psychometric, neurological, and electroencephalographic comparisons. *American Journal of Psychiatry, 127*(5), 634–645.

Wilens, T. E., Faraone, S. V., Biederman, J., & Gunawardene, S. (2003). Does stimulant therapy of attention-deficit/hyperactivity disorder beget later substance abuse? A meta-analytic review of the literature. *Pediatrics, 111*(1), 179–185.

Woodward, L. J., Fergusson, D. M., & Horwood, L. J. (2000). Driving outcomes of young people with attentional difficulties in adolescence. *Journal of the American Academy of Child and Adolescent Psychiatry, 39*(5), 627–634.

Xu, C., Reid, R., & Steckelberg, A. (2002). Technology applications for children with ADHD: assessing the empirical support. *Education and Treatment of Children, 25*(2), 224–248.

Yang, P., Chung, L.-C., Chen, C.-S., & Chen, C.-C. (2004). Rapid improvement in academic grades following methylphenidate treatment in attention-deficit hyperactivity disorder. *Psychiatry and Clinical Neuroscience, 58*, 37–41.

Young, S., Bramham, J., Gray, K., & Rose, E. (2008). The experience of receiving a diagnosis and treatment of ADHD in adulthood. *Journal of Attention Disorders, 11*(4), 493–503.

Zalecki, C. A., & Hinshaw, S. P. (2004). Overt and Relational Aggression in Girls With Attention Deficit Hyperactivity Disorder. [References]. *Journal of Clinical Child and Adolescent Psychology, 33*(1), 125–137.

NOTES

1. Pharmaceutical advertising is the exception I have in mind.
2. *See* Chapter 1.
3. These would typically be called "sequelae," but that term tends to reify ADHD, which is something I would like to avoid; *see* section on reification.
4. This scale was developed by Lenard Adler, Ronald C. Kessler, and Thomas Spencer; Accessed 9/12/07 from http://www.med.nyu.edu/psych/assets/adhd-screen18.pdf.
5. ADD (attention deficit disorder) is an older term for ADHD. The term is still sometimes used for the inattentive subtype of ADHD; Hallowell and Ratey use it to refer to all subtypes of ADHD.
6. Intervention usage and availability vary widely, but the trend in recent years is "toward increased use of medication and decreased intensity of psychotherapeutic visits" (Leslie & Wolraich, 2007, 110).
7. The AAP's guideline and the AACAP's 2007 practice parameter address treatment of school-aged children with ADHD; AACAP's 2002 practice parameter concerns use of stimulant medications more generally but is directed primarily at ADHD therapy. (American Academy of Child and Adolescent Psychiatry, 2002; American Academy of Pediatrics, 2001; Pliszka et al., 2007)
8. At least, this is the case in the predominant view. Those who object to medicalization generally, or to medication in particular, may reject the transition. For example, one criticism of medicalization is that it encourages a falsely easy way

out of distress, both for the affected individual and for the larger society. It is "too easy" for the individual because of its implied excuse of responsibility; "too easy" for society because the individual, rather than society, needs to do most of the adjusting. *See* section "The Drug Wars and Skeptics' Intolerance."
9. Recommendation 10 reads: "If a patient with ADHD has a robust response to psychopharmacological treatment and subsequently shows normative functioning in academic, family, and social functioning, then psychopharmacological treatment of the ADHD alone is satisfactory" (Pliszka, et al., 2007, 912).
10. To what extent adults' "acceptance" stage (Young et al., 2008) equates to the structuring of self in children (Singh, 2007) is an open question.
11. *But see* Chapter 2 about the lack of data supporting long-term efficacy of treatment.
12. For more discussion of the ongoing controversies, *see* Chapters 1 through 3.
13. Some of the concern is for safety: This medical issue is discussed briefly in Chapter 1.
14. The antipsychiatry claims of the Church of Scientology, in particular, are disreputable enough that even Thomas Szasz distances himself from them; these I give no more attention.
15. McHugh mentions attention deficit disorder (in adults), post-traumatic stress disorder, obsessive-compulsive disorder, and social phobia as examples of psychiatrically defined disorders that are better conceived as matters of individuality (McHugh, 1999).

6 NEW DIRECTIONS

If the analysis so far is right, our medical, scientific, and cultural practices interact to accidentally reinforce intolerance of ADHD-diagnosable people. The seemingly obvious solution—simply confront the intolerance!—certainly deserves a try. So does challenging any rhetoric or action that promotes one-sided benefits, such as drug-company profits or a researcher's career. But because the intolerance is normalized, deeply embedded in goals and assumptions of ubiquitous systems, and constantly reinforced, tackling the roots of the problem might prove more effective.

To clarify this overarching goal, "reducing intolerance" is not the same as "increasing tolerance." "Increasing tolerance" reflects an underlying attitude that there is something wrong about which one is tolerant. The goal of reducing intolerance requires a deeper change in perspective, a shift in how much human variation we can recognize not as something to be "tolerated" but simply as how people are.[1] This shift, emphatically, does *not* mean abandoning care or closing off options for anyone, and it equally emphatically embraces scientific knowledge. But it does mean that we, jointly, need to establish new approaches.

Change in perspective and action is urgently needed. This book describes ADHD as understood under DSM-IV, depicting practices in vogue through 2012 (American Psychiatric Association, 2000). But revised criteria in the DSM-5 suggest little that solves problems raised in earlier chapters (American Psychiatric Association, 2013). In fact, the new DSM-5 criteria up the ante. They add symptoms, especially subjective and behavioral criteria relevant to adults, pulling additional behavioral, emotional, and subjective experiences under the banner of "disorder." The new criteria may also increase the prevalence of diagnosed ADHD in other ways, adding to the steep growth over the 2000s.[2] The potential for more diagnoses arises because the new criteria lower the bar from requiring "impairment" to requiring "negative impact"; increase the number of subjective symptoms; increase the age at first symptoms from 7 to 12 years, so that those whose symptoms develop during grade school or early middle school would become diagnosable; and decrease the minimum number of symptoms needed for adult diagnoses from six to five. Without change in our approaches to ADHD, then, it is likely that we will simply direct intolerance to more people.

To avoid that result, we need to change two aspects of practice. First, we need a framework—what I will call the Pragmatist framework—for deciding what actions to take, and assessing whether a given approach to ADHD has been or can be both ethically *and* epistemically successful.[3] The section that follows establishes this framework, explaining and justifying my recommendation (Recommendation 1) that decisions about ADHD that have public relevance need to more carefully take both facts and values into account. (The framework can be adapted to making determinations about other medical or medicalized conditions.) Second, using the Pragmatist framework, we need to determine what specific ADHD-related medical, scientific, and social practices are likely to achieve both ethical and epistemic success. I offer three recommendations for change (Recommendations 2–4). With respect to these three recommendations, I recognize that I cannot anticipate or represent the diverse expertise and interests needed to determine the direction and effective means of change. Nor can I predict the many unknowns in funding, scientific theories of ADHD, future social needs, and efficacy of new approaches. For these reasons, my recommendations are fairly general, although I offer concrete examples in the section "The Recommendations in Practice." The aim, overall, is that the four recommended changes work together to make progress toward widely shared goals: reducing intolerance, increasing knowledge, and offering appropriately tailored care and resources to ADHD-diagnosable people.

Recommendation 1. Establish a Pragmatist Framework That Carefully Uses Facts *and* Values in All Decisions and Actions Relevant to ADHD

Changing approaches to ADHD without repeating mistakes requires choosing a new direction and determining how to avoid past errors. To do this requires articulating the goals—that is, to establish what ends we *value* and what errors we deplore. It also requires determining how to reach the goals—the means—which requires *facts*. In this section, I offer first a rationale for the first recommendation, then a practical strategy for implementing it. The argument, although brief and necessarily incomplete, derives from the writings of American Pragmatist John Dewey, improved by insights from feminist philosophers of science, especially Helen Longino. Briefly, the way forward is to move past stale controversies, and to redirect attention to action—that is, to the need to choose what to *do*—keeping facts, values, and their enmeshment in view.

Both public and private decision making can benefit from progress toward the first recommendation. I focus, though, on public decisions of broad reach, such as determining what research to fund, what disorders the DSM includes, or what drugs or other interventions are "safe" and "effective." Such decisions affect many—sometimes millions—of people, including anyone who directs policy, studies or treats ADHD, teaches or parents diagnosed students, is diagnosable him/herself, or who interacts with a diagnosable person. Basic principles of fairness suggest that those affected should have a voice—somehow—in making such judgments. Yet a worry immediately arises that opening debate to those affected will simply raise a cacophony of conflicting opinions. This concern is important, given decades of disagreements, and true consensus among those affected is unlikely. But common ground does exist to motivate work on improving approaches to ADHD. For example, the affected millions share a need to provide or to take advantage of affordable medical care, teaching, and learning. Most people also endorse the importance of raising happy and successful children; supporting everyone's freedom to pursue their own goals, whether or not affected by ADHD; and improving knowledge of ADHD through scientific research. Despite the multiple disagreements detailed in earlier chapters, some shared or overlapping interests and values provide a basis for progress.

Rationale for the Pragmatist Framework

Earlier chapters showed that people consistently *do* draw on facts and values in their individual, social, medical, and scientific reasoning about ADHD. (The traditional division between facts and values says, roughly, that "facts" are information that has already been empirically demonstrated, whether by scientific procedures or less formal observation; "values" are, again roughly, the broad class of ethical stances and practical interests. I will show later that facts and values cannot be so clearly compartmentalized.) Parents, for example, typically consider both facts and values when deciding whether their child should take stimulant medications. They might consider facts about efficacy and side effects—in general and in their own child's case—and goals they value for their child (Chapter 5). Psychiatrists establishing diagnostic criteria consider facts about frequencies and clustering of behaviors, and values concerning what constitutes an impairment (Chapter 1). Scientists choosing hypotheses or endpoints (Chapters 2 and 4), teachers and clinicians setting their individual standards for referral or diagnosis (Chapter 3), or individuals opting to seek diagnosis (Chapter 5) also typically consider facts and values. But most people do this tacitly, rather than thinking carefully about the justification and relevance of the facts and values their actions or arguments imply. Tacitly drawing on facts and values has led to the automatic association of "ADHD" and "bad" in clinical, educational, social, individual, and scientific reasoning. In turn, as we have seen, accepting the association accidentally reinforces intolerance. It has also, via continuous reinforcement of DSM-defined ADHD, contributed to a relative stasis in scientific gains (Chapter 4). As discussed further below, learning instead to use facts and values *explicitly and critically* will help change this pattern.

The first recommendation also helps overcome several persistent obstacles to change. The first obstacle is multiple disagreements over *specific* (purported) facts, values, or combinations of fact and value (specific as opposed to general disagreement about the relevance of facts as a class, or values as a class; *see* discussion of "trumping," below). For example, Chapter 5 describes the tenacious hold of a debate over medication use in which parties differ over specific values: One side embraces psychopharmaceutical use as an aid, the other decries it as coercive. The second obstacle is intransigence, in the name of an identified fact or value, or for the sake of an unnamed interest, need, or demand for power or influence. Certainly intransigence shores up some struggles for allies and dominance described in Chapter 3. The third obstacle is lack of resources for achieving desired goals. I will address these three barriers in the course of discussing the fourth, which is to base decision making on two mistaken assumptions: that facts and values *are* dichotomized, and that they *should* be.

The two mistaken assumptions pervade most decisions and debates surrounding ADHD. Yet, contrary to the first assumption, earlier chapters showed that existing facts surrounding ADHD are not value-free, nor are existing values fact-free. Instead, facts and values intertwine in current medical, scientific, educational, and social knowledge and practice. When we nevertheless assume that facts and values are dichotomized, we fail to recognize practical realities. This failure can then obfuscate or distort decision-making. For example, if people fail to recognize that economic (and other) values contribute to the DSM's categorical model of ADHD (*see* Chapter 1), they risk importing the embedded black-and-white needs of resource allocation—determining that some people get ADHD treatment and some do not—into judgments that require complex, shades-of-gray thinking. This risk of error might be enough to steer people from the mistake, but there are also good reasons to think that the dichotomization assumption is unwarranted not just practically speaking, and not just for the case of ADHD, but generally.[4] This further claim questions the second assumption—that facts and values *should be* dichotomized.

People often refer to the (supposed) fact/value dichotomy as the gap between "is" and "ought," using Hume's terminology (Hume, 1978 [1740]). The gap can be interpreted logically, metaphysically (pertaining to what exists), or epistemically (pertaining to what is known). Those who endorse the logical interpretation claim that it is a fallacy to derive a statement of the form "women *ought* to be beaten" from a statement of the form "women *are* beaten." In this simple form, Hume's point is unassailable, and arguments that make such illicit moves fail (miserably, in the example). But the simple form misses two features of language and practice. First of all, one can, by degrees, build legitimate arguments that move from "is" to "ought." For example, one can argue for a first premise, "If there is intolerance, we ought to prevent it," citing both facts about the results of intolerance and values that establish the need for prevention. Adding the second premise "There *is* intolerance of ADHD-diagnosable people," one can then soundly conclude that "We *ought* to prevent intolerance of ADHD-diagnosable people."[5] More centrally, however, the first premise relies on a common feature of our language and thought, the use of a thick ethical term, "intolerance." This term already embeds, in its meaning, both facts and values. (*See* Chapter 4 for a discussion of how thick ethical terms embed values in the scientific literature.) It thus, in effect, provides a pivot point that allows the transition from is to ought. Relying on a thick ethical term does not introduce a logical flaw, although the term's contents require close examination.

A metaphysical interpretation of the fact/value dichotomy is, very roughly,[6] that "facts" pertain to entities that exist physically (by taking up space, for example), whereas "values" pertain to human preferences and to the qualities of individual, singular experiences. Values, in such a view, have a nonphysical existence, like ideas or concepts. But Dewey objects that our world does not compartmentalize into an "inside" and "outside." In the one world we have, human experiences and preferences are as concretely part of that world as solid objects are.

The metaphysical noncompartmentalizing extends to epistemology, too. The traditional claim is that facts are objective, and values are subjective.

However, in Dewey's terms, experience is interactive, engaged, participatory, and mutually influential—the world acts on us, shaping the subjective impressions that contribute to our knowledge and our values, and we act on the world, coming up against it and altering it. This mutual influence makes the subjective/objective boundary porous, and along with it, the fact/value boundary. In addition, continues Dewey, most reasoning, including most scientific reasoning, is practical[7] —the point of reasoning is to choose what to *do* (Dewey, 1998 [1915]). Practical reasoning involves a series of judgments. Some judgments are relatively more descriptive, some more practical. *Descriptive judgments* assess an object or situation—"the given"—without acting on it; they tend to be oriented to the past or present. One might, for example, survey the literature and determine that "Aspirin relieves headaches." Such descriptive judgments equate roughly to facts (Hume's "is"); they commonly, but not necessarily, refer to "outer" ("objective") considerations. Potentially, they contribute to understanding the *means* to a goal (headache relief, in this case). *Practical judgments* direct action toward a particular *goal* (the "oughts") and thus tend to be oriented to the future. *Value judgments,* says Dewey, are a species of practical judgment, directed toward making changes that bring about good or mitigate bad.[8] They commonly, but again not necessarily, refer to "inner" ("subjective") considerations. One might judge, for example, that it would be good to get rid of one's headache, and then draw on the descriptive judgment about aspirin to supply the means. Both descriptive and practical judgments are hypotheses, not determinate; both have truth conditions that may or may not be met.[9] Thus, epistemically, too, is's and oughts, facts and values can be roughly distinguished but not compartmentalized (*see also* Chapter 4 and Putnam, 2002). Those who assume that fact and value should be dichotomized confuse these rough distinctions for dichotomies. This confusion *invents* absolute logical, metaphysical, and epistemological barriers to considering facts and values, goals and means, subjective and objective, and the rest, in the same scale—but these absolute barriers do not exist.[10]

Recognizing the porousness makes it easier to see two consequences relevant to ADHD. The first, which this book has emphasized, is that values influence the facts of clinical science.[11] The second—less discussed so far—is that facts influence values. Contrary to the common myth that values are immune to reason, people often change their values with changing circumstances and knowledge (Anderson, 2004). For example, a person might cease to value corporate climbing if the effort made her miserable, or abandon her preference for a food when she developed an allergy to it. People learn, with effort, to abandon prejudices; among these might be prejudices that disadvantage people who are ADHD-diagnosable. In Deweyan terms, we are capable of adjusting our goals, as well as our means.

These issues might seem esoteric, but dichotomization of facts and values has practical effects. It distorts discussion of choices, because under the assumption, people cannot understand the full content of value-laden facts or fact-laden values. Some of the contentiousness around ADHD derives from the resulting confusion. Denying the assumption that facts and values ought to be dichotomized can help clear the disagreements—or at least clarify the grounds of disagreement. Even clarifying the grounds for disagreement helps overcome the first persistent obstacle to change, the disagreements over specific facts and values, by isolating the point of contention. For example, people disagreeing over ADHD drug prescriptions might agree on what the drug does, but not on whether that action benefits users. Or they might disagree that an effect has been demonstrated, while sharing a goal.[12]

Dichotomization also gives people in power a tool—the trumping strategy—to strengthen their position. The trumping strategy varies according to aims and audience. The first step is always to size up an audience to determine whether it favors facts (or particular facts) or values (or particular values). The strategist can then declare facts generally, values generally, or a particular fact or value their trump card. For example, drug industry representatives, when speaking to scientists and clinicians, assume that the audience favors facts. They then present their research and its conclusions as pure fact, even when these are designed to promote their own values, such as interest in profit. Tobacco companies and anti-environmentalist groups have mastered a variation (Oreskes & Conway, 2010). They frequently pretend to favor fact-seeking, but disingenuously distract the audience by endlessly contesting facts—this gains them time to pursue valued ends, such as profit and political gain. Others choose to trump with values generally or with a specific value. This may require ignoring facts (or ignoring other values), at least selectively. For example, those who oppose psychopharmaceutical use on principle may choose not to hear evidence that favors drug use for some individuals. Similarly, those who prioritize low-cost treatment, parsed in economic terms, will deny the relevance of facts about higher-cost alternatives. Such strategies earn their users a reputation approvingly termed "principled" and disapprovingly called "dogmatic." Yet another maneuver indirectly promotes a trumping fact by exploiting the assumption that values are fact-free. The strategist argues, in effect: Because values are uninfluenced by facts, basing decisions on values is unreasonable (or emotional, hysterical...). So hardheaded members of the audience (scientists, business people, policy makers) should ignore claims based on value judgments. Typically, in the ADHD case, this strategy paints scientists and their clinical partners as truth-bearers and deems critics or skeptics the truth-deniers blinded by values. Frequently, though, the strategists are not themselves scientists or clinicians but people with other agendas, such as profit or redirection of resources.

These trumping strategies often effectively silence critics. Part of the effectiveness derives from the relative power of the person or group using such maneuvers. Part, though, depends on the audience accepting the trumping. If audiences instead recognized the need to consider facts, values, and their overlap, they could more readily resist the ploys. Progress toward the flexibility of carefully considering facts and values, goals and means—the Pragmatist framework—could then make headway against the persistent obstacle of intransigence.

Implementing the Pragmatist Framework

Let's get more concrete about how a new Pragmatist framework for decision making would work in practice. To review, the problem at hand is that the current practice of tacitly blending fact and value in investigation, practice, and debate surrounding ADHD has resulted in intolerance and, very likely, slowed the growth of knowledge (*see* Chapter 2, page 65). Attempting to solve this problem by dichotomizing facts and values misrepresents both in-practice and theoretical relationships between facts and values. The goal, instead, is to establish a framework that will let people carefully use facts *and* values in all decisions and actions relevant to ADHD. Broadly, the path I propose, drawing on Dewey, is to redirect practices of investigation, practice, and debate to the need to choose what to *do*—to action. In this mode, acts of practical judgment, rather than isolated facts or values, become the primary, nondichotomized category, dispelling the trump-inspiring gap between facts and values.

But who will be using the Pragmatist framework? As we have seen, large numbers feel the consequences of decisions about research agendas, medical and education access, intervention emphases, and other far-reaching choices. The idea that public input is needed in complex cases that blend medicine, science, and policy has been voiced by many philosophers (e.g., Douglas, 2009; Kitcher, 2011; Kourany, 2010; Longino, 1990). Dewey, with great faith in people and in democratic principles, would argue for a radically democratic approach, without concern about reaching any predetermined results. But, whatever its appeal, the ideal of inclusiveness tends to give way, in practice, to power politics, impracticality, and other issues. Feminists have long noticed the dearth of women's voices in science and politics; other voices are readily squelched also—those of the poor, disempowered races or ethnicities, children, the ill or disabled. These concerns are crucial here, as many of those affected by ADHD are among the disempowered, and practical issues, such as resource availability, also loom. So how, in practice, would this large and diverse group of people provide considered and effective input?

Although the need to take action would also help maintain focus on an issue, institutions would clearly need to streamline the process. For example, adequate representation would have to substitute for direct input. Equally clearly, decision makers would not be able to reach a conclusion on every facet of every issue. They could only set up a workable procedure, and do their best to judge the evidence, air the range of views, and prioritize the considerations on the table—despite knowing that facts, values, and priorities would change with time. Procedures would be unique to each institution, and I will not attempt to address the details here. Each, though, would need to meet the initially stated guidelines for the Pragmatist framework: (1) The focus would be on deciding what to do, and (2) Those involved would need to recognize that facts and values are both relevant to these decisions.

More guidelines would be needed, however. To avoid abuses and distortions, no trumping would be allowed. People would instead need to argue in favor of facts and values. Given other safeguards on the debates (see below), well-justified facts and values would not be overturned in such discussions. However, an admittedly troublesome precondition for non-trumping also needs to be established: decision makers would need to be willing to change their views in the face of evidence. In the case of ADHD, all parties would, at the very least, need to give up dogmatic conceptions of ADHD or of anti-ADHD commitment.[13]

In addition, effective procedures would need safeguards against two other problems: the problem of powerful groups or individuals who can sidetrack or undermine thoughtful decision making (intentionally or not) and the problem of uninformed and easily swayed popular opinion. Longino (1990, 2002) has provided safeguards to protect scientific knowledge against these problems, thereby increasing its degree of objectivity. Broadened, and with some important amendments, Longino's safeguards prove useful for action-oriented decision making in broader communities as well.

Longino's four safeguards for enhancing objectivity are that the community (again, she is referring specifically to scientific communities, while I am broadening her points) establish venues for criticism; exhibit uptake of the criticism; base discussion of criticism on public, shared standards; and recognize tempered equality of intellectual authority (Longino, 1990, 76–80; Longino, 2002, 131–134). The first of these, establishing venues for criticism, makes seeking alternative viewpoints a required part of decision-making processes. Within scientific communities, for example, peer review is one such venue. But peer review can be overly insular, as when like-minded peer reviewers favor their pet theories. Longino argues for avenues that value criticism from a wide range of perspectives. Ideally, having such avenues would provide a structure for all relevant voices to receive a hearing. Many practical decision-making institutions already have some pathways available. But, as with peer review, improved procedures in political, educational, medical, and other venues could build on existing ones.

The existence of avenues for criticism is not enough to ensure uptake of justified criticisms or concerns, however. Longino's uptake requirement insists that knowledge-generating communities be appropriately responsive to criticism—and that the critics be similarly responsive. Adapted to the groups making ultimate decisions about ADHD—for example, the Work Groups writing the DSM, administrators setting school policy, or medical boards settling on standards of care—the uptake requirement insists that the groups actually be receptive to criticisms and concerns. The criterion does not automatically require that the decision-makers change course, but it does require defending the chosen course against relevant critique and changing course if the defense fails. At the same time, critics—whether their critique stems from disagreements on facts or values—also need to drop or amend their arguments as appropriate.

Despite the importance of considering a wide range of criticisms, expertise does play a central role in furthering scientific knowledge. Expertise often provides perspectives and a grasp of possibilities and impossibilities that non-experts cannot develop. Recognizing this, as well as the varying intellectual capacity among individuals, Longino amended her original third criterion—"equality of intellectual authority" (Longino, 1990, 78–79)—to recommend tempered equality of intellectual authority (Longino, 2002, 131–132). Longino's tempering allows that some do not have the intellectual capacity to engage in scientific knowledge making. It also allows a distinction between *intellectual* authority (widely shared capacities for reasoning, communication, and other rational activity) and *cognitive* authority (the specific expertise that helps scientists recognize, for example, the relative certainty of hypotheses about a phenomenon).

When broadening Longino's recommendation to wider decision making, two basic points remain: not everyone can fully engage, and expertise is important. But these points need to be understood differently in the context of public decision-making.[14] First, procedures must sharply increase the *number* of people considered capable of relevant input. Although such proposals raise worries about uninformed opinion misdirecting policy, Elizabeth Anderson argues that the worries are misguided, expanding on Dewey's point that "'the cure for the ailments of democracy is more democracy'" (Anderson, 2011, 157). Anderson provides criteria by which laypersons can readily analyze the content and strength of scientific claims.[15] This argument and procedure help allay some concerns. But ADHD-relevant decisions involve children, whose capacities for analyzing science have not yet developed, as well as some adults for whom Anderson's procedures would be out of reach. Some form of inclusion or representation must also let their voices be heard. Second, it is crucial to recognize that with a complex, lived phenomenon like ADHD, many *different types* of experts can provide input that others, including non-experts, cannot. Depending on the choice at hand, expertise in medicine, science, education, administration, public policy, public health, parenting, or lived experience might be the most crucial. Each form of expertise would require tempering, from time to time, by the expertise of the others. Although no formula for achieving this goal exists, meeting the criterion at a minimum requires careful attention to and respect for others' expertise.

To have a reasonable debate at all, as opposed to mud-slinging or exercises of power, *some* principles or procedures must be held fixed. Longino argues that public, shared standards are needed for criticism and response. For the scientific communities Longino discusses, those standards are scientific, counted on to generate scientific knowledge. For public debates focusing on decision-making the standards will differ. At base, these include the standards discussed above—focusing on action, recognizing the relevance of both facts and values, and disallowing trumping. Other standards are also critical to reasoned debates, particularly those that help people weight facts and values by standards of merit, and those that help people determine the relevance of varying criteria. Articulating these standards is difficult, of course, and too much for this space. The goal, though, would be to keep the standards minimal, so that they could be more inclusive. In addition, as Longino and Dewey both argue, the standards themselves need to be open to criticism and revisable.

Admittedly, recommending this Pragmatist framework, and the considered use of facts and values, requires optimism. For starters, the practical procedures would require much effort in streamlining and prioritizing. In addition, the recommendation itself does nothing to solve one persistent obstacle to change—limited resources. To make the effort and any investment of resources seem worthwhile, those involved would need to keep the shared goals in mind—wanting and needing "good" approaches to ADHD, in all the rich epistemic, ethical, and practical senses of that word. Progress toward implementing the Pragmatist framework also has the added benefit that it works against the other obstacles to change. It localizes and clarifies disagreements, contributing to their solution. It removes possibilities for obfuscation that allow dogmatism or ulterior motives to masquerade as expertise or virtue, and it of course models non-dichotomization, improving practices of debate and decision making going forward.

The next three recommendations aim at more specific areas of practice around ADHD, although like the first they have application to other issues in clinical science, and perhaps beyond.

Recommendation 2. Avoid Dichotomizing

Early chapters argued that the ubiquitous practice of grouping individuals into "ADHD" and "non-ADHD" categories, although useful for distributing resources, also segregates a group toward which many people direct intolerance. Non-dichotomizing practices, in contrast, encourage people to think and act in terms of complex individuals, rather than in terms of groups or types. As with attending to individuals in other stigmatized groups (races, genders, sexualities), attending to ADHD-diagnosable individuals helps people notice individual strengths and character, apart from group-associated traits. Recognizing individual variation complicates the understanding of ADHD, decreasing the tight association with "badness." The goal of the second recommendation, then, is that people establish non-dichotomizing practices that will contribute toward greater inclusiveness and less intolerance.

One concrete step toward this goal is to stop reifying ADHD. Rather than thinking and acting as if ADHD were a permanent, definitive, biological feature of individuals, practices would reflect the fact that, at present, ADHD is a hypothetical and pragmatic construct, like "intelligence" or "kindness," at least as much as it is a biological difference. Anyone—parents, teachers, clinicians, diagnosed individuals, journalists, and others—can change their perspective and actions. But it can be difficult to do so when the reified view is the norm. Although people typically understand that their children, students, patients, and themselves are complex and unique, labels and categories can still narrow their angle of vision, shaping their attitudes in accord with the category. It takes practice and support from others to maintain a perspective in which ADHD-associated traits are only some among many characteristics the diagnosable individual possesses.

Because of their expertise and influence, clinical scientists and psychiatrists would take the lead in encouraging this change in perspective. Experts' individual conversations and public rhetoric would consistently convey a non-reified view, so that the altered understanding could filter to clinicians, educators, and the public (for more on the clinical scientists' role, see Recommendation 3). Coupled with research to determine the effectiveness of new strategies (Recommendation 3), schools, primary care physicians, and mental health clinicians could also take practical steps toward individualization by modifying diagnosis and interventions.[16] In general, professionals could focus diagnosis and interventions for ADHD-associated difficulties less to the broad-strokes category "ADHD" complicated by "comorbidities," and direct attention instead to specific, practical individual impediments to individually endorsed goals. Already, in practice, clinicians recognize that ADHD is a "grab-bag" diagnosis, but they could more carefully consider the consequences of fitting diverse individuals into a single pattern. In a potentially important move in this direction, the DSM-5's Section III includes "cross-cutting" dimensional assessments (American Psychiatric Association, 2013). These assessments allow clinicians to systematically track impairment in various general measures of function and well being (such as sleep, mood, and substance abuse) across categories rather than within the confines of a specific mental disorder. Such assessments could encourage attention to individual circumstances. With care in implementation,[17] such changes could contribute to reaching the second goal.

In addition, interventions could also draw on specific, practical individual strengths. Precedents for such approaches exist. For example, some schools currently practice "differentiated" education. Teachers using these methods tailor classroom activities to students with varying needs, including differences in interests, culture, preparation, and general ability, in addition to medically identified variations. Directing more funding to studying and supporting effective approaches might increase the useful options. Notably, individualized approaches could also address concerns of ADHD-diagnosable adults who need to adapt their home or workplace environments or schedules to their own strengths and weaknesses. Depending on the person, individualized adaptation might mean, for example, a quieter workspace or a faster-paced home life or job.

The systemic changes needed to avoid dichotomization would likely require policy changes and reallocation of resources. For example, if standards shifted, procedures and systems that rely on today's standardized diagnosis and treatment would likely lose out. Such changes might conflict with the interests of drug companies, current clinical practice and insurance systems, many educational systems, and scientific research framed in today's standards. Change, then, would require broad support from those who would benefit from it. Ideally, the inclusive Pragmatist framework would help secure the changes.

Recommendation 3. Study New Disease Models and Forms of Intervention

Study of mental function and mental disorders has helped develop options to relieve distress. Progress in science has also altered, but not eliminated, judgmental attitudes toward mental disorders (Chapters 4 and 5). But with changes in their research programs—particularly, reducing dependence on DSM classification, attending more to within-group variation, and increasing emphasis on non-pharmaceutical interventions—clinical scientists could simultaneously add knowledge about mental disorders, consider new options for those affected, and contribute to reducing intolerance. Social influences on all aspects of science, from the choice of questions investigated to financial and professional rewards, mean that changing the goals and procedures of scientific research are not solely scientists' responsibility. Nevertheless, scientists could often take the lead.

Basing the overwhelming majority of mental health research on DSM categories has systematized research and facilitated conversation across disciplines (Chapter 2). But narrowing the bulk of studies to this pattern has also reinforced negative epistemic, practical, and ethical consequences (Chapter 4). To reduce dependence on the DSM categories, scientists could more often design studies using existing alternative models of ADHD, such as dimensional and biopsychosocial models (Chapter 1), and they could more often entertain novel hypotheses. In addition, more emphasis on investigating typical and variant function in areas such as attention, learning, memory, and physical activity—as opposed to the focus on studying specific disorders—would offer ample research space for developing new questions. Shifting study toward a broader range of interests would allow a more pluralistic, less reductionistic, and less dichotomized search for causes, mechanisms, and interventions—assuming funding followed suit.

The methodological change of attending more often and in more detail to variation within groups, rather than taking group averages as adequate representations, would likely verify considerable diversity among those who have

ADHD (Chapter 2). Recognizing this diversity, in turn, could help decrease dichotomized thinking about ADHD, a step toward redressing the tight associations between "bad" and "ADHD" (Recommendation 2). Like going beyond the DSM, this methodological change could also contribute to knowledge. For example, researchers could seek and untangle the sources of diversity among the myriad interactions of mind, body, environment, relationships, time, development, and individual variation.

Opening new avenues for research could also have considerable practical impact. Earlier chapters have discussed the decades-long emphasis on pharmaceutical interventions, and the relative dearth of behavioral, educational, or novel interventions for ADHD. By revealing only a subset of the available facts, such emphases close off potential solutions by default, while new questions could lead to new interventions. In particular, looking ahead to the next recommendation, researchers could question the assumption that the environment cannot be significantly changed, and direct more research toward environmental effects. Opening investigation in this direction might lead to new interventions, or even to prevention.

Scientists studying pharmaceuticals could also head in new directions. For example, there is a dearth of long-term data on treatment efficacy. Studying long-term effects might, or might not, verify the strong intuition and personal experience of many that drug therapy for ADHD improves lives in the long run. Part of the new direction, however, needs to be refined definitions of "efficacy" that accurately reflect the successes prized by ADHD-diagnosed individuals. This point brings us back to Recommendation 1—the need to consider both facts and values. A new understanding of "efficacy" needs to attend equally to facts such as the ecological validity of measures chosen to assess it, and the values embedded in the chosen measures (*see also* Chapters 1, 2, and 4).

The move to a more pluralist science, like changes from decreased dichotomization, has "winners" and "losers." Research funding patterns would need to change: at least relatively speaking, funding for study of ADHD as a problem solved primarily by drug use would decrease, while funding for new avenues would increase. This could not simply *happen*, however. Those served by science's investigations—parents, clinicians, teachers, and diagnosable individuals, as well as the scientists involved—would need to lobby for research likely to benefit them or people in their care (Recommendation 1). Conversely, research—and scientists—could benefit from seeking out and addressing a wider set of needs.[18] If promising new avenues did arise from early research, social support could grow. Such change would mark a new alliance (Chapter 3).

Recommendation 4. Focus Less on Changing Individuals, More on Changing Society

As earlier chapters have explained, the predominant view of ADHD localizes ADHD's dysfunctions within individuals. Focusing on individual pathology leaves social contributions to "disorder" and social contributions to its relief underexamined. For example, rather than considering the possibility that work or school expectations are unrealistic, and therefore changing the expectations, people persuaded by the predominant view seek to change individuals to meet the goals. An assumption at work here—that the social structure cannot be changed, or at least not significantly changed—often strengthens people's commitment to intervening at the individual level. The assumption is sometimes true, of course—necessity may dictate that we make decisions in accord with the social structures we, or those for whom we are responsible, live in. Teachers, clinicians, and parents have to act in high-pressure environments that offer limited support and time. Diagnosable individuals have to determine their choices now, not in an idealized world. But that does not mean that social change is impossible or impractical in every situation. After all, we made considerable shifts in research, clinical care, and social support for ADHD over the past 30 years. Why not—given adequate study—make changes that would avoid the intolerance embedded in today's ADHD constructs?

Some social interventions are relatively simple, and we have precedents. Biopsychosocial models of disease often look for straightforward cultural or structural changes that can decrease or even dissolve the impact of disabilities (World Health Organization, 2002) (*see* Chapter 1). For example, although our society has a long way to go in terms of full access for all, we do provide structures such as elevators, sidewalk ramps, and lower drinking fountains, allowing people with a broad range of abilities to access buildings and activities. In the case of ADHD, simple changes like putting a diagnosed child's desk near the teacher's is already accepted practice. With changes in emphasis and funding (Recommendation 3) researchers could seek similar minor, but effective, alterations. Future studies, together with social support (Recommendation 1), might even support more extensive structural change. For example, perhaps smaller class sizes, or allowing more movement in classrooms, or building more vigorous physical activity into the school day would benefit *all* students, not just ADHD-diagnosable ones. Adults' needs require similar attention.

The goal of changing social expectations is more amorphous and difficult than simple structural interventions; it is also more contentious, as it contrasts varying sets of values. Proposing this goal also immediately raises the question, "Changing social expectations to what?" Determining the "what" once again requires careful, public examination of the relevant values and facts—the goals and the means to reach them (Recommendation 1). For example, ADHD-diagnosed people are said to be less successful than non-diagnosable people by standard measures of academic achievement and income. But should current social mores about "success" stand? What careers and lifestyles should count as successful? Should we continue to accept the forms of testing, accommodation, and credentialing we now value in academics and the workplace—forms that disadvantage some people? What expectations realistically draw on people's strengths, and work around their weaknesses? Many educators, disability rights activists, parents of ADHD-diagnosed children, or diagnosable adults might propose new perspectives. The same groups might lead outreach and public education to stimulate the commitment to social change. At the same time, scientists and clinicians could determine which changes make empirical sense (Recommendation 3). In the end, the currently predominant choice of standard diagnosis and treatment might win out, but, at present, alternatives deserve consideration.

The Recommendations in Practice

How might the recommendations work, in practice? And how might they build on each other? The following examples give the basics on a few currently contentious issues. Experts and stakeholders in each venue have the knowledge and interests needed to work out the details.

In Medicine

Many public debates center on the question, "How should we spend our money?" Allocating medical resources for ADHD-diagnosable people is no exception. Decisions about resource allocation affect millions of people, directly or indirectly—for example, diagnosable people and their contacts, clinicians in various specialties, and insurers and the insured. To follow the Pragmatist framework, decision makers would establish a procedure to gain input from all these voices. They would consider facts, such as the number of dollars and other resources available, the expertise of clinicians, the efficacy of interventions, and the physiological features of individuals. They would also consider and debate the values that establish spending priorities. For example, they would discuss the extent to which the medical system should offer options in addition to the predominant form of management (diagnosis, drug treatment), given individual and family preferences; consider the opportunity costs of spending money to solve problems associated with ADHD, rather than on some other health issue; and debate how various priority rankings would support or detract from the goal of reducing intolerance.[19]

In this picture, the four recommendations each get a hearing, and may work together. Those making the decisions would be using the Pragmatist framework to prioritize both facts and values. The resulting discussions would include consideration of the other recommendations as well: whether continued dichotomizing is appropriate, or new research is needed, or whether some currently medicalized problems might more fruitfully be considered social issues.

In Science

Research funding, too, is a matter of public interest. As we have seen, ADHD research to date has heavily emphasized the search for biological mechanisms located within individuals, along with investigation of drug interventions. In large part, funding choices drive this emphasis. The large percentage of ADHD research funded by the pharmaceutical industry is presently out of public control, and I will not discuss here how to manage the resulting skewing of the research agenda (Chapter 4).[20] But government institutions, such as the National Institutes of Health (NIH) or publicly funded universities, could adopt more inclusive decision procedures, given that citizens ultimately provide the funding.

Current NIH funding procedures emphasize facts, such as findings of previous research, the feasibility of the proposed research, and demonstrations of efficacy from related studies. The procedures also recognize values relevant to the funding choices, such as the ethics of the proposed study, and the projected practical or ethical significance of the work. However, in the picture I am proposing, the time and expertise devoted to the second aspect of grant applications would need greater emphasis, given the complexity of the issues. Just some of the values in play include judgments of the "significance" of one project relative to another—weighing a project based in neuroscience versus one in developmental psychology, perhaps; judgments as to what counts as "progress"; and priorities for future healthcare expenditures driven by the research. Adequate attention would require more robust and inclusive input on these (and other) values than is typical of today's decisions, so that consensus decisions could take the rich range of considerations into account.

Once again, the four recommendations work together: implementing the Pragmatist framework that prioritizes both facts and values (Recommendation 1) sets the stage for progress on other goals, by at a minimum raising the possibility of changed research priorities (Recommendation 3) that might decrease dichotomization (Recommendation 2) and contribute to social change (Recommendation 4).

In Education

One educational issue ripe for public discussion concerns the goals we set for children. Current expectations for behavior, attention, and achievement correlate with today's 11% (Centers for Disease Control, 2012) ADHD prevalence among children and adolescents. Some reports suggest that high expectations directly contribute to high diagnostic rates, rather than simply correlating with them. For example, stimulant prescriptions among the youngest children in a classroom, who would tend to be at a developmental disadvantage in meeting expectations, are nearly double that of the older students (Elder, 2010). Do the younger children really have ADHD at twice the rate, or are classroom expectations simply too high for many children at their age level? If expectations are too high, *which* expectations—behavioral, academic, or other—need amendment? Similarly, the push to extend ADHD into preschool years and even toddlerhood raises important questions about the choice to pathologize common behaviors of very young children.

To discuss these issues, decision makers would need to identify the values underlying goals for children, as well as facts about children's capacities. Debates would draw in other values as well, including views on classroom atmosphere and teacher support, and attitudes toward the relative risks of diagnostic labeling versus potential underserving of ADHD-diagnosable children. Among the many additional facts for decision makers to consider would be what resources are available to reach desired goals and what consequences follow for diagnosable people who are diagnosed and for those who are not. The need to develop data to help guide potential social change shows once more the interlinking of the chapters' recommendations.

Educators have already established groundwork for implementing the Pragmatist framework to debate the possibility of change: many decisions about funding and school structure already require input from those affected by a given decision, alongside relevant research.[21] Refined procedures would increase efforts to reach those affected, avoid sway by powerful factions, and prevent trumping of facts by values, and vice-versa.

Conclusion

Accidental Intolerance has traced the multiple strands—medical, scientific, and social—that tightened into the predominant ADHD concept and into today's attitudes and practices. I have proposed that we can, jointly, change our practices to dispel the intolerance we accidentally ended up with. We can do this by implementing the Pragmatist framework, which guides us to carefully consider facts and values whenever we make decisions relevant to ADHD. I anticipate, as well, that we would choose to curtail dichotomization, open new branches of research, and opt, more often, for social change. Fortunately, given the complexity of these recommendations, substantial grounds for agreement on goals already exists, particularly across a broad middle range that recognizes pros and cons of various approaches and perspectives, rather than asserting extreme views.

Perhaps change could even be broader, as in some ways ADHD is not unique. Mutually influential medical, scientific, and social phenomena also marginalize many others who have clinically defined conditions. Among the many subject to intolerance are people who have other psychiatric disorders, such as depressive disorders or social anxiety; those affected by the so-called "functional disorders," such as fibromyalgia and chronic fatigue syndrome; and those affected by "lifestyle" conditions, such as obesity, substance abuse, or addiction. Although some solutions will be unique to each condition, my four recommendations, suitably adapted, offer a means toward progress on these other fronts as well.

REFERENCES

American Psychiatric Association (2000). *Diagnostic and Statistical Manual of Mental Disorders* (4, Text Revision ed.). Arlington, VA: American Psychiatric Association.

American Psychiatric Association (2013). *Diagnostic and Statistical Manual of Mental Disorders: DSM-5* (5th ed.). Washington, DC: American Psychiatric Association.

Anderson, E. (2004). Uses of value judgments in science: a general argument, with lessons from a case study of feminist research on divorce. *Hypatia*, 19(1), 1–24.

Anderson, E. (2011). Democracy, public policy, and lay assessments of scientific testimony. *Episteme*, 8(2), 144–164.

Arras, J.D. (2001). Freestanding pragmatism in law and bioethics. *Theoretical Medicine and Bioethics*, 22(2), 69–85.

Brendel, D. H., & Miller, F. G. (2008). A plea for pragmatism in clinical research ethics. *The American Journal of Bioethics*, 8(4), 24–31.

Centers for Disease Control and Prevention (2012). 2011–2012 National Survey of Children's Health. Retrieved April 12, 2013, from http://www.cdc.gov/nchs/slaits/nsch.htm.

Chai, G., Governale, L., McMahon, A. W., Trinidad, J. P., Staffa, J., & Murphy, D. (2012). Trends of outpatient prescription drug utilization in US children, 2002–2010. *Pediatrics, 130*(1), 23–31.

Clough, S. (2003). *Beyond Epistemology: A Pragmatist Approach to Feminist Science Studies.* Lanham, MD: Rowman and Littlefield.

Dewey, J. (1998 [1915]). The Logic of Judgments of Practice. In L. A. Hickman, Alexander, Thomas M. (Ed.), *The Essential Dewey: Volume 2: Ethics, Logic, Psychology* (pp. 236–271). Bloomington and Indianapolis, IN: Indiana University Press.

Douglas, H. E. (2009). *Science, Policy, and the Value-Free Ideal.* Pittsburgh, PA: University of Pittsburgh Press.

Elder, T. E. (2010). The importance of relative standards in ADHD diagnoses: evidence based on exact birth dates. *J Health Econ, 29*(5), 641–656.

Fins, Joseph J., Bacchetta, Matthew D., & Miller, Franklin G. (1997). Clinical Pragmatism: a method for moral problem solving. *Kennedy Institute of Ethics Journal, 7,* 129–145.

Goldenberg, M. J. (2009). Iconoclast or Creed?: Objectivism, Pragmatism, and the Hierarchy of Evidence. *Perspectives in Biology and Medicine, 52*(2), 168–187.

Hume, D. (1978 [1740]). Book III: Of Morals; Part I: Of Virtue and Vice in General; Section 1: Moral Distinctions Not Deriv'd From Reason. In P. H. Nidditch (Ed.), *A Treatise of Human Nature* (pp. 469). Oxford, UK: Oxford University Press.

James, W. (2011 [1907]). Pragmatism's Conception of Truth. In R. B. Talisse, Aikin, Scott F. (Ed.), *The Pragmatism Reader: From Peirce Through the Present* (pp. 79–91). Princeton, NJ: Princeton University Press.

Kincaid, H., Dupre, J., & Wylie, A. (Eds.). (2007). *Value-Free Science? Ideals and Illusions.* Oxford, UK: Oxford University Press.

Kitcher, P. (2011). *Science in a democratic society.* Amherst, NY: Prometheus Books.

Kourany, J. A. (2010). *Philosophy of Science after Feminism.* New York: Oxford University Press.

Lacey, H. (1999). *Is Science Value Free? Values and Scientific Understanding.* New York: Routledge.

Longino, H. E. (1990). *Science as Social Knowledge: Values and Objectivity in Scientific Inquiry.* Princeton, NJ: Princeton University Press.

Longino, H. E. (2002). *The Fate of Knowledge.* Princeton, NJ: Princeton University Press.

Machamer, P., & Wolters, G., eds. (2004). *Science, Values, and Objectivity.* Pittsburgh, PA: University of Pittsburgh Press.

Oreskes, N., & Conway, E. M. (2010). *Merchants of doubt : how a handful of scientists obscured the truth on issues from tobacco smoke to global warming* (1st U.S. ed.). New York: Bloomsbury Press.

Peirce, C. S. (2011 [1878]). How to Make Our Ideas Clear. In R. B. Talisse, Aikin, Scott F. (Ed.), *The Pragmatism Reader: From Peirce through the Present* (pp. 50–65). Princeton, NJ: Princeton University Press.

Putnam, H. (2002). *The Collapse of the Fact/Value Dichotomy and Other Essays.* Cambridge, MA: Harvard University Press.

World Health Organization (2002). *Towards a Common Language for Functioning, Disability, and Health: ICF: The International Classification of Functioning, Disability, and Health.* Geneva: World Health Organization.

NOTES

1. To the extent that variation is simply variation, "tolerating" differences is really a sign of irritability—something for *tolleraters,* not the *tolerated,* to work on.
2. ADHD medication prescriptions increased 46% between 2002 and 2010 (Chai et al., 2012), indicating a similar increase in diagnostic rates (*see* Chapter 1).
3. Others have also proposed approaches to clinical and medical ethics, and/or to clinical science, that are based on American Pragmatism (e.g., Fins, 1997; Arras, 2001; Clough, 2003; Brendel 2008; Goldenberg, 2009). Detailing the similarities and differences among these efforts and the framework I propose is beyond the scope of this project. One element of difference, however, is the extent to which they are bidirectional, in the sense of applying equally to facts and values—or, to speak in terms of practical fields, to clinical science and clinical- and bioethics. A second is the extent to which the theorist's understanding of Pragmatism is "freestanding" versus metaphysically committed.
4. Generally, that is, for facts not true by definition, or according to set rules. I do not claim, for example, that mathematical facts embed values; *see also* endnote 6.
5. In fact, this book makes such an argument.
6. Full discussion of scientific and moral realisms and antirealisms is beyond the scope of this book.
7. c. f. endnote 4. The exception is reasoning that relies solely on definitions and internally consistent rules. These allow "controlled inferences," by exempting the object of inference from interaction and change. (Dewey, 1998 [1915], 267)
8. I am doubtful that values are necessarily a form of *judgment*. Some are, such as sophisticated tastes in wine or food. Others, such as valuing relief of hunger, seem to be noncognitive but nonetheless foundational for choosing goals. This point requires much more discussion.
9. Pragmatists, as is well known, do not understand truth, or truth conditions, in an absolute sense. Peirce's definition of truth gives one version: "The opinion which is fated to be ultimately agreed to by all who investigate, is what we mean by the truth, and the object represented in this opinion is the real" (Peirce, 2011 [1878], 63). James' definition gives another: " 'The true', to put it very briefly, is only the expedient in our way of thinking, just as 'the right' is only the expedient

in our way of behaving. Expedient in almost any fashion; and expedient in the long run and on the whole, of course; for what meets expediently all the experience in sight won't necessarily meet all farther experiences satisfactorily. Experience, as we know, has ways of *boiling over*, and making us correct our present formulas" (James, 2011 [1907], 86–87).
10. Dewey concentrates on one consequence of breaking down the fact/value, objective/subjective dichotomy, concluding that value judgments are objective (again, in a nondichotomized sense). However, many other theorists since Dewey have taken up the other consequence, arguing that judgments of fact are importantly subjective—underdetermined, theory laden, with values embedded, and so forth. (Chapter 4). The prior discussion has shown that this is the case for facts derived from clinical science. But Dewey shows us why, more generally, imperfectly objective science is not inherently a problem, although it does require a new approach to scientific reasoning, and reasoning about science.
11. The influence of values on science has been the topic of much discussion in recent philosophy of science. Longino's work, cited later, has been very influential. Other contributions to this discussion include Douglas (2009); Kincaid, Dupre, and Wylie (2007); Lacey, (1999); and Machamer and Wolters, (2004).
12. Agreements and disagreements could, of course, be much more fine grained than in this rough example.
13. Some will find the precondition troublingly idealistic. There are, of course, similar preconditions—and potential problems—for *any* public discussion that attempts to be both reasoned and open.
14. Longino notes that this issue will arise (Longino, 2002, 133).
15. Other roadblocks to engagement, she argues, do need to be addressed for public policy making to be effective. These include biased reporting, people's segregation in like-minded groups, and "cultural cognition" that leads people to overrate factual claims that agree with their own biases (Anderson, 2011).
16. These steps overlap with the goal of considering both facts and values. Part of what needs to be thought about in establishing new approaches and their efficacy is to consider and critique the values packed into the terms "pragmatic" and "effective." What achievements are necessary for individuals and for society? Which are desirable? How might we measure efficacy in terms of economic and human results? Educators, physicians, psychologists, sociologists, ethicists, activists, and others would have much to contribute in addressing such questions.
17. Because the DSM-5 continues to define ADHD as undesirable, increased focus on individuals, without additional changes, will likely not be enough to undo intolerance. For example, the approach could backfire if looking at additional aspects of diagnosable people's lives allowed more circumstances or choices to be perceived as symptomatic. This result would add more negative associations with ADHD, strengthening its valence (*see* Chapters 3 and 4).

18. Thank you to Kristen Intemann for this point.
19. Issues would arise, as well, in which facts and values were difficult to disentangle. For example, both facts and values, as we saw in Chapter 1, contribute to views on what conditions may properly be described as "medical," versus "idiosyncratic," freely chosen, social, legal, spiritual, or some other designation.
20. Private control limits the role for influential input from a wide range of sources—although, given that input represents consumers, industry *might* take an interest in novel opportunities presented by those dissatisfied with the status quo—assuming there was profit to be made on the ideas.
21. The initial decision to include ADD/ADHD as a disability for the purposes of special education, for example, was based on widespread input and a survey of relevant research.

INDEX

AACAP (American Academy of Child and Adolescent Psychiatry), 134, 152, 157, 173*n*7
AAP (American Academy of Pediatrics), 17, 134, 173*n*7
Abrams, S.J., 100
acceptance of individuals, 159–160
accidental intolerance, 142–174
    about, 142–143
    byproducts of practice, 151–156
    drugs and skepticism of, 163–165
    perspectives on ADHD, 143–151
accommodation plan, development of an, 82–83
accumulated difference, dichotomization and, 61–62
action, focus on, 177, 182, 185
actor-network theory (Latour), 8, 111–112*n*1, 112*n*2
ADD (attention-deficit disorder), 25, 82, 113*n*19, 173*n*5
    See also ADHD (attention-deficit hyperactivity disorder)
Adderall (amphetamine, dextroamphetamine mixed salts), 15, 90, 118, 148
ADHD (attention-deficit hyperactivity disorder)
    1970s adjectives used to describe, 144–145*t*
    2000s adjectives used to describe, 144*t*
    about, 1–11
    alternative models, 26–37
    animal models for, 54–55
    biological aspect of, 3
    current view of, 37
    defined, 14
    diagnosis of, 14–15
    differences in perspective of, 1–2
    DSM-IV-TR diagnostic criteria for attention-deficit hyperactivity disorder, 4–5*t*
    DSM-5 diagnostic criteria for attention-deficit hyperactivity disorder, 175–176
    history of, 24–26
    initial causes of, 15
    in medicine, 13–38, 43–45
    perspectives on, 1–2, 143–151
    prevalence of ADHD, 13
    research on, 47, 58–61
    types of, 14–15, 26
    uptake of, 162–163
ADHD: diabetes analogy, 152

ADHD-diagnosed children and adults, as allies, 85–86
ADHD science, shaping, 46–78
  about, 46
  reasoning patterns, 47–57
  structure by choice, 57–70
ADHD science, values in, 115–141
  about, 115–117
  assumptions, 123–125
  constitutive values, 129–135
  containable bias, 117–118
  context, 125–129
  core methodology, 129–135
  feedback loop, 135–136
  investigative trends, 118–123
  language, 125–129
  questions, 123–125
Adler, Leonard, 173n4
"Adult ADHD Self-Report Scale," 147
adversaries. *See* destabilizers and adversaries
advocacy groups
  as allies, 91–92
  viewed as destigmatizing force, 97
African-Americans, 101, 148
allies
  ADHD-diagnosed children and adults as, 85–86
  advocacy groups as, 91–92
  parents as, 84–85, 113n12
  pharmaceutical companies as, 90–91
  physicians as, 86–89
  psychologists as, 87
  science as, 92–94
ambivalence, of individuals, 159–160
American Academy of Child and Adolescent Psychiatry (AACAP), 134, 152, 157, 173n7
American Academy of Pediatrics (AAP), 17, 134, 173n7
American College of Obstetrics and Gynecology, 17

American Pragmatism, 196n3
American Psychiatric Association, 3, 13, 149
amphetamine, dextroamphetamine mixed salts. *See* Adderall
analogy
  animal model: human "link," 54–55
  reasoning by, 76n6
Anderson, Elizabeth, 129, 131, 185
animal models, for ADHD, 54–55
assumptions, in feedback, 123–125
atomoxetine (Strattera), 90–91, 120
attention-deficit disorder (ADD), 25, 82, 113n19, 173n5
  See also attention-deficit hyperactivity disorder (ADHD)
attention-deficit hyperactivity disorder (ADHD)
  1970s adjectives used to describe, 144–145t
  2000s adjectives used to describe, 144t
  about, 1–11
  alternative models, 26–37
  animal models for, 54–55
  biological aspect of, 3
  current view of, 37
  defined, 14
  diagnosis of, 14–15
  differences in perspective of, 1–2
  DSM-IV-TR Diagnostic Criteria for Attention-Deficit Hyperactivity Disorder, 4–5t
  history of, 24–26
  initial causes of, 15
  in medicine, 13–38, 43–45
  perspectives on, 1–2, 143–151
  prevalence of ADHD, 13
  research on, 47, 58–61
  types of, 14–15, 26
  uptake of, 162–163
averages, in ADHD science, 62–64

backtracking, 77n9
Barkley, R.A., 67, 78n27, 147
Bechtel, William, 55–56, 59–60, 75n3, 76–77n8, 77n12
bias, 117–118, 120, 141n8
biased reporting, 197n15
Biederman, J., 114n24, 117–118
biological models, of mental disorders, 20
biological perspective
  on ADHD, 3, 17
  of ADHD research, 47, 58–61
  as byproduct of practice, 152–153
  social perspective vs., 36
biopsychosocial models
  of disease, 190
  of mental disorders, 20
Boorse, Christopher, 27–28
Breggin, Peter
Talking Back to Ritalin, 163
Brown Attention-Deficit Disorder Rating Scale, 16
buproprion (Wellbutrin), 120
Burns, M.K., 114n29
Bussing, R., 101

candidate genes, 69, 78n28
"Capturing America's Attention" report, 148–149
Castellanos, F.X., 78n27, 128
categorical concepts
  complicating, 68–69
  dimensional concepts vs., 31–33
categorical dimensions, 44n13
categorical model, scientific inaccuracies of, 32
CDC (Centers for Disease Control), 92
CHADD (Children and Adults with Attention-Deficit/Hyperactivity Disorder), 91–92, 97, 99, 114n28

Chesapeake Institute of Washington, D.C., 121
Church of Scientology, 174n14
Ciba Pharmaceutical Company, 90
clinical focus, 61
clinicians, fact and value considerations of, 178
cognitive authority, 184
cognitive-energetic model (Sergeant), 78n27
Cohn, Howard, 90
Colombo, A., 44n8
community control groups, 132
comorbidity, 20, 63, 64, 112n6, 153
Computer Retrieval of Information on Scientific Projects (CRISP), 92–93
Concerta, 148
concomitant diagnosis, 112n6
Conrad, P., 34–35, 45n19
constitutive values, 129–135
constraints, on individuals, 156–157
containable bias, 117–118
context, in feedback, 125–129
convergence, 53–54
core methodology, 129–135
Craver, C.F., 76–77n8, 77n9
CRISP (Computer Retrieval of Information on Scientific Projects), 92–93
cross-cutting dimensional assessments, 187
cross-sectional methods, 141n8
cross-sectional MRI, 130
"cultural cognition," 197n15
cultural consensus, 150

Danforth, S., 149–150
Darden, L., 76–77n8, 77n9
default mode hypothesis (Castellanos and Sonuga-Barke), 78n27
descriptions, of an object, person, event, or phenomenon, 125

descriptive category of research, 47–48
descriptive judgments, 180
descriptive studies, 76n7
destabilizers and adversaries
    about, 94–95
    equity as, 99
    ethnicity as, 101–102, 114n30
    gender as, 103
    imperfect translation as, 95–98
    race as, 101–102, 114n30
    testing as, 100–101
deviance, 22, 35, 45n18
Dewey, John, 177, 180–181, 182, 185, 197n10
diagnosis
    of ADHD, 14–15
    concomitant, 112n6
    potential for, 175–176
    psychodynamic vs. organic
        approaches to, 44–45n17
    rates of, 1–2, 30–31, 44n8
Diagnostic and Statistical Manual of Mental Disorders. See DSM *(Diagnostic and Statistical Manual of Mental Disorders)*
diagnostic criteria
    for ADHD (DSM-IV-TR), 4–5t
    for ADHD (DSM-5), 175–176
    DSM, 22–26
    judgments in, 44n14
    used as an operationalization, 52–53
dichotomization
    accumulated difference and, 61–62
    anti-medicalizers objections to, 98
    avoiding, 186–188
    as byproduct of practice, 152–155
    categorical models and, 33
    of control groups, 132
    of facts and values. See fact/value dichotomy
    Lyman on, 141n13
    methodological commonness of, 141n9
    observation of differences and, 64–65
    power of, 181
    statistical analysis and, 133
difference, described, 29–31
Diller, Lawrence, 100–101, 157–158
dimensional assessments, cross-cutting, 187
dimensional concepts, categorical concepts vs., 31–33
dimensional models, 33
Dimoska, A., 127, 128
"discrete kinds," 31
disease
    about, 18
    biopsychosocial models of, 190
    categories of, 14
    Hawthorne on, 29
    value-free notion of, 27
    value-ladenness of, 29
DNA replication, 75n2
DNA sequences, patterns in, 123
dopamine, 119–120
drug companies/industry
    about, 98
    as allies, 90–91
    research funded by, 117, 148, 192
    role in publicizing messages, 148
drugs
    about, 36–37
    amphetamine, dextroamphetamine mixed salts (Adderall, Adderall XR), 15, 90, 118, 148
    atomoxetine (Strattera), 90–91, 120
    buproprion (Wellbutrin), 120
    debate over use of, 178
    global sales of, 43n5
    methylphenidate (Ritalin), 15, 25, 90, 119, 163
    prescriptions for, 114n24, 196n2
    proponents of, 164
    rates of, 44n8
    scientists studying, 189
    skepticism of, 163–165

DSM *(Diagnostic and Statistical Manual of Mental Disorders)*, 3, 13, 119
DSM-II, 24
DSM-III, 25, 82, 84
DSM-III-R, 25–26
DSM-IV, 26, 53, 175
DSM-IV-TR, 4–5t, 26
DSM-5, 26, 33, 65, 175–176, 187, 197n17
DSM model
  key debates, 56–57
  of mental disorders, 22–24
  scientific inaccuracies of, 32
  studying the syndrome described by, 78n21
Dumit, Joseph, 78n25
Durston, S., 54, 63–64, 130, 131, 141n8
dynamic developmental theory (Sagvolden et al.), 78n27
dysfunction
  anti-medicalizers attributions of, 98
  as byproduct of practice, 152
  described, 28–31
  Hawthorne on, 29
  scientific judgment of, 28
dysfunctional behavioral inhibition model (Barkley), 78n27

education, recommendations in, 193
Education, U.S. Department of, 121
effectiveness, 113n23, 132, 197n16
efficacy, 113n16, 113n23, 132
Eisenberg, Leon, 86
Elliott, C., 90, 158
emotional disturbance, special educational category of, 101–102
endophenotypes, 68, 78n26
environmentalists, 164
environmental precursors, 17
equity, as an adversary, 99
eradication, critics on, 97
ERIC database, 140n5

ethnicity
  as an adversary, 101–102, 114n30
  stereotypes of, 148
etiological hypotheses, 57, 58
etiology, static view of ADHD's, 131
excessive bias, 120

facts
  construction of, 111–112n1
  cultural meanings, incorporated in, 123–124
  defined, 177
  Pragmatist framework, use in, 176–186
fact/value dichotomy, 26, 178–179
  arguments against, 115–136, 179–182
  practical effects, 181–182
Faraone, Stephen, 117–118
feedback, 115–141
  about, 115–117
  assumptions, 123–125
  constitutive values, 129–135
  containable bias, 117–118
  context, 125–129
  core methodology, 129–135
  feedback loop, 135–136
  investigative trends, 118–123
  language, 125–129
  questions, 123–125
feedback loop, 135–136
feminists, 129–130, 182–183
findings, defined, 50–51
'fledgling psychopaths,' 146
fMRI (functional magnetic resonance imaging), 55, 128
forward chaining, 77n9
Fulford, K.W.M., 29, 44n8
functional magnetic resonance imaging (fMRI), 55, 128
future directions, 175–198
  about, 175–176
  Recommendation 1: Pragmatist framework, 176–186

future directions (*Cont.*)
　Recommendation 2: Avoid dichotomizing, 186–188
　Recommendation 3: Studying new disease models and forms of intervention, 188–189
　Recommendation 4: Changing society, 190–191
　recommendations in practice, 191–193
"fuzzy kinds," 31

Gannett, L., 123–124, 125
gender, 103, 147–148
generalizations
　based on averages, 134
　framing of as reasoning pattern, 48–49
　misunderstanding of, 149
　scientists on, 148
　scope of, 75*n*2
　of structure, 62–69
Glennan, S., 76–77*n*8
goals
　normalization of, 164
　varied fields with unifying, 47

Haack, Susan, 53–54
Hacking, Ian, 160–161
Hallowell, E.M., 150, 173*n*5
harmful dysfunction analysis, of mental disorder, 28–29
Haslam, Nick, 31–32, 33, 36, 44*n*15
Hawthorne, Susan, 29
healthcare expenses, 17
"Healthy People 2010" initiative, 97
"Healthy People 2020" initiative, 97
Hispanics, 101
human behavior, medicalization of, 159
Hume, D., 179
hyperactivity/impulsive-type ADHD, symptoms of, 15, 175–176

hyperkinesis, 82, 143
hyperkinetic impulse disorder, 144–145*t*
hyperkinetic reaction of childhood, 24–25
hypothesis, defined, 50–51

IDEA (Individuals with Disabilities Education Act) (2004), 83–84, 99, 114*n*28
IEP (individualized education program), 82–83
impairment, 87
imperfect translation, as an adversary, 95–98
inattention, 15
inattentive-type ADHD, symptoms of, 15, 175–176
'increasing tolerance,' 175
individualized education program (IEP), 82–83
individuals
　acceptance of, 159–160
　ambivalence of, 159–160
　constraints on, 156–157
　effects of ADHD on, 156–163
　fact and value considerations of, 178
　relief of, 159–160
　social pressures on, 157–159
Individuals with Disabilities Education Act (IDEA) (2004), 83–84, 99, 114*n*28
inhibitory control, 140–141*n*7
insurance coverage, 87
intellectual authority, 184
intelligence tests, 131–132
interlevel reasoning, 49–52
internalizing, by individuals, 160–162
intervention
　about, 97
　in future, 187
　literature about, 140*n*5
　in schools, 81–84, 121

studying, 122
  usage and availability of, 173n6
intransigence, 178
invariance, standards for, 49
investigative trends, 118–123

James, W., 196–197n9
Jensen, P.S., 147, 152
Journal of Attention Disorders, 121
judgments
  descriptive, 180
  in diagnostic criteria, 44n14
  of dysfunction, 28
  normative, 146
  practical, 180
  value, 44n12, 180, 196n8

Karatekin, C., 55
Kessler, Ronald C., 173n4
Kraepelin, Emil, 44–45n17
K-SADS (Kiddie Schedule for Affective Disorders and Schizophrenia), 16
Kuhnian paradigm, 78n22, 119

labeling, 96, 114n29
language, in feedback, 125–129
Latour, Bruno
  actor-network theory, 111–112n1, 112n2
  on Pasteur, 94
  recruiting allies, 92
  translations, 89
line drawing, 29–31
Lister, Joseph, 76n6
Longino, H.E., 124, 177, 183–185, 197n11
long-term correlates of ADHD diagnosis, 149
Lunbeck, Elizabeth, 44–45n17

Machamer, P., 76–77n8, 77n9
McHugh, Paul, 159, 164, 174n15
McNeil Pharmaceuticals, 148

mechanisms, 44n10, 55–56, 59–60, 76–77n8
mechanism schema, 77n9
mechanism-seeking category of research, 47–48
mechanism sketch, 77n9
mechanistic studies, 76n7
medical concepts, 14–22
medicalization
  of human behavior, 159
  objections to, 173–174n8
  social perspective *vs.*, 34–36
medication
  amphetamine, dextroamphetamine mixed salts (Adderall, Adderall XR) 15, 90, 118, 148
  atomoxetine (Strattera), 90–91, 120
  buproprion (Wellbutrin), 120
  debate over use of, 178
  methylphenidate (Ritalin), 15, 25, 90, 119, 163
  prescriptions for, 114n24, 196n2
  proponents of, 164
  rates of, 16–17, 31, 44n8, 84–85, 101, 103, 157, 196n2
  scientists studying, 189
medicine, shaping ADHD, 13–45
  about, 13–14
  alternative models, 26–37
  medical concepts, 14–26
  recommendations for, 191–192
Medline database, 140n5
mental disorders
  biopsychosocial models of, 20
  DSM Model of, 22–24
  harmful dysfunction analysis of, 28–29
  Hawthorne on, 29
  history of, 19–20
  medical model of, 21–22
  psychodynamic models of, 19, 20
mental illness, 27

methylphenidate (Ritalin), 15, 25, 90, 119, 163
minimal brain dysfunction
   as ADHD precursor, 143
   common diagnosis of, 82
Mostofsky, S.H., 130, 131, 141n8
MTA (Multimodal Treatment of ADHD trial), 88, 133, 134–135

NAMI (National Alliance on Mental Illness), 91–92, 97
National Association of State Directors of Special Education, 99
National Comorbidity study, 20
National Education Association, 99
National School Boards Association, 99
"natural kinds," 31
Navarro, V., 149–150
negative terminology, 146
negative valence, 149
neuronal, 75n1
neuroses, 24
neuroticism, 31
The New England Journal of Medicine, 90
NIH funding, 192
non-Hispanic blacks, 101
non-Hispanic whites, 101
"non-kinds," 31
norepinephrine, 120
normal control groups, 132
normalization
   goal of, 164
   rates of, 133
normative judgments, 146
"no significant difference," 68
nosology, 22

OHI (other health impairment) category, 83, 101, 112n7, 112n8, 112n10, 112n11
operationalization, 52–53, 132
operations, 44n10

oppositional defiant disorder, 67, 78n23
organic approaches, to diagnosis, 44–45n17
organic brain syndrome, 25
other health impairment (OHI) category, 83, 101, 112n7, 112n8, 112n10, 112n11

parents
   as allies, 84–85, 113n12
   fact and value considerations of, 177–178
pattern-seeking, 123–124
Peirce, C.S., 196–197n9
personality disorders, 24
perspectives
   on ADHD, 1–2, 143–151
   biological, 36, 47, 58–61, 152–153
   social, 36
pharmaceutical companies/industry
   about, 98
   as allies, 90–91
   research funded by, 117, 148, 192
   role in publicizing messages, 148
pharmaceuticals. *See* drugs
pharmaceutical treatment, 154, 157
pharmacological approaches, 122
pharmacotherapy, 17, 98
physical entities, 58–59
physicians
   as allies, 86–89
   involvement of, 113n15
Pliszka, S.R., 128
positive feedback loop, 136
practical judgments, 180
"practical kinds," 31
practical reasoning, 180
practice
   byproducts of, 151–156
   recommendations in, 191–193
pragmatics, 60–61, 196–197n9, 197n16
Pragmatist framework

about, 176–177
  implementing the, 182–186
  rationale for, 177–182
prescription medication, 114n24, 196n2
prevalence of ADHD, 13, 31, 83, 101
primary care physicians, 15–16
psychiatrists, fact and value considerations of, 178
PsychINFO database, 140n5
psychodynamic approaches, to diagnosis, 44–45n17
Psychodynamic Diagnostic Manual (PDM), 32
psychodynamic models
  about, 32, 33
  of mental disorders, 19, 20
psychologists
  as allies, 87
  involvement of, 113n15
psychoses, 24
Public Health Service, 97
Putnam, H., 125

race
  as an adversary, 101–102, 114n30
  stereotypes of, 148
Ratey, J.J., 150, 173n5
reasoning patterns, 47–57
  analogy, 54–55
  convergence, 53–54
  generalizations, 48–49
  interlevel reasoning, 49–52
  key debates, 56–57
  mechanism, 55–56
  operationalization, 52–53
  types of studies, 47–48
  varied fields with unifying goals, 47
recommendations
  Avoid dichotomizing, 186–188
  Changing society, 190–191
  in practice, 191–193
  Pragmatist framework, 176–186

Studying new disease models and forms of intervention, 188–189
reducing intolerance, 175
reductionism, 58–61
Rehabilitation Act (1973), 112n5
reification
  of an ADHD type, 70
  as byproduct of practice, 155–156
  error of, 53
reinforcement, consistent, 142
relief, of individuals, 159–160
research
  in ADHD, 47, 58–61
  categories of, 47–48
  funded by pharmaceutical companies, 117, 148, 192
  intervention, 122
  recommendations for, 188–189
Ritalin (methylphenidate), 15, 25, 90, 119, 163
Rouse, Joseph, 93
Rubia, K., 54–55, 120

Sagvolden, T.
  on dopamine, parenting styles and cultural expectations, 66, 76n5, 120
  dynamic developmental theory, 78n27
  interlevel theory, 51–52
Satterfield, J.H., 53
schema instantiation, 77n9
schizophrenia, 44–45n17
Schneider, J.W., 34–35, 45n19
schools, intervention in, 81–84, 121
Schwartz, P.H., 30, 44n12
science
  as an ally, 92–94
  influence of values on, 197n11
  recommendations for, 192–193
science shaping ADHD, 46–78
  about, 46
  reasoning patterns, 47–57
  structure by choice, 57–70

science, values in ADHD research, 115–141
  about, 115–117
  assumptions, 123–125
  constitutive values, 129–135
  containable bias, 117–118
  context, 125–129
  core methodology, 129–135
  feedback loop, 135–136
  investigative trends, 118–123
  language, 125–129
  questions, 123–125
scientific fields, varied with unifying goals, 47
scientists, fact and value considerations of, 178
Scientology, Church of, 174n14
scope, standards for, 49
Section 504, 83–84, 112n5
segregation, in like-minded groups, 197n15
sequelae, 173n3
Sergeant, J., 78n27
serotonin, 120
Shire Pharmaceuticals, 90, 118, 148
short-term behavioral control, 122
Singh, I., 95–96, 160, 161
SNAP scale, 53, 113n16
social allies and adversaries, 79–114
  about, 79–80
  allies, 81–94
  destabilizers and adversaries, 94–104
social perspective
  biological perspective vs., 36
  medicalization vs., 34–36
social pressures
  as byproduct of practice, 154–155
  on individuals, 157–159
Sonuga-Barke, E.J.S., 78n27
special education services, 112n11, 114n29
Spencer, Thomas, 173n4

standardized admissions tests, 100
stasis, 65–66, 69
statistics
  Adderall sales in UK, 90
  ADHD patients to patient load ratio, 16
  biological focus, 47
  children treated by 1970, 25
  cost of ADHD care, 87
  cost of treatment in MTA, 88
  diagnosis rates, 30–31, 113n13
  educational expenses, 83–84
  education services, 112n11
  gender, 103
  healthcare expenses, 17
  medication prescriptions, 16–17, 31, 44n8, 84–85, 101, 103, 157, 196n2
  mental disorders, 20
  office visits in 1998, 43n3
  prevalence of ADHD, 13
  race/ethnicity, 101–102, 114n30
  research grants, 93
stimulant medication
  as most common form of treatment, 15
  See also medication
Strattera (atomoxetine), 90–91, 120
stress-diathesis models, 20
structure by choice, 57–70
  about, 57–58
  biological focus, 58–61
  dichotomization and accumulated difference, 61–62
  generalization, 62–69
  reductionism, 58–61
  reification, 70
studies, types of, 47–48
Szasz, Thomas, 34, 163, 164

teachers, fact and value considerations of, 178
testing, as an adversary, 100–101

Thagard, Paul, 76*n*6
therapeutic category of research, 47–48
thick ethical terms, 125
Timimi, Sami, 34, 164
"tolerating" differences, 196*n*1
tractability, 60–61
traits, 144–145*t*
transient situational disturbances, 24
traveled paths, 66
treatment
   efficacy of, 189
   most common form of, 15
   See also medication
trends, investigative, 118–123

United Kingdom, diagnosis and medication rates in, 44*n*8
United States
   clinical trials of drugs, 114*n*27
   diagnosis and medication rates, 44*n*8
U.S. Department of Education, 121

value judgments, 44*n*12, 180, 196*n*8
value laden, 140*n*2
values
   constitutive, 129–135
   controversies over, 94–104

defined, 43*n*1, 177
in disease or disorder models, 27–33
functioning like facts, 29
influence on science of, 115–136, 197*n*11
in medical practice, 14
in social conception of ADHD, 79–94
values in ADHD science, 115–136, 140–141
   about, 115–117
   assumptions, 123–125
   constitutive values, 129–135
   containable bias, 117–118
   context, 125–129
   core methodology, 129–135
   feedback loop, 135–136
   investigative trends, 118–123
   language, 125–129
   questions, 123–125
value valence, 140*n*2

Wakefield, J.C., 28–29, 44*n*11
Wellbutrin (buproprion), 120
Williams syndrome, 31–32
Woodward, L.J., 68
Work Groups, 184